How to Talk Dirty

Over 101 Dirty Talk Examples to Spice up Your Sex Life

Andrew King

Table of Contents

Introduction

Congratulations on downloading How to Talk Dirty and thank you for doing so!

The following chapters will discuss the art and science of dirty talking, because yes, it is both of these things. You will learn some helpful tips for getting you into the game and learning how to use that mouth of yours in an entirely new way.

Why learn to talk dirty? Well, for starters, it intensifies your sex life and makes everything much hotter. There is no downside to telling your partner what they're doing right and just how hot they are. The science proves it; a 2012 study published in the *Journal of Social and Personal Relationships* found that the more comfortable we are talking about sex, the better the sex.

Dirty talk can be intimidating. It can be scary. It can be awkward. Read these words;

Yeah, baby, right there, you're so hot.

It reads a bit ridiculous, right? Just the idea of saying that out loud to another person is weird to think about.

The reality is, the majority of us love to hear dirty talk in the bedroom (and if you're one of these people who aren't, there's something for you too in this book!) After all, who wouldn't want to hear about how hot they are to their partner?

In this book, we will cover exactly the reasons why dirty talk is so important, dos and don'ts, and best of all, 101 phrases to help you get started.

There are plenty of books on this subject on the market, so thanks again for choosing this one! Every effort was made to ensure it is full of as much useful information as possible. Please enjoy!

Chapter 1: The Basics, and What Is Dirty Talk

So, really, what is dirty talk?

Dirty talk is the act of speaking to another person in a sexual manner, with the goal of making the person feel sexually aroused.

There are several different terms for it, including, sexy speak, naughty talk, erotic whispers, filthy nothings, the list goes on. Call it whatever you are comfortable with. The goal always remains the same. To get some.

But why do we like dirty talk? Why is it so awkward? Why does it feel so taboo and naughty?

It really comes down the sexiest part of our entire body - our brains. Your brain is where every dirty thought, every filthy fantasy comes from, so when you think about it, it actually makes sense. Your brain is what decides what's attractive to you, what you like and don't like. It decides what gets you going and what slams on the breaks. This is actually just one of many, many areas where men and women are different.

In your mind, there is something called a hypothalamus, and in it are two different parts - the preoptic area and the suprachiasmatic nucleus area. They have their own unique uses, for men and women. The preoptic area is the area of your mind that is directly related to mating, is more than two times bigger in men, and has twice more cells. The suprachiasmatic nucleus, on the other hand, specializes in reproduction cycles and is different in size between men and woman. For women, it is elongated, and for men, it is shaped like a sphere.

This explains a lot, doesn't it? It really all boils down to sex drive. Men have more testosterone, so that means their sex drive is higher than women's. There's even a difference between what women want to hear and what men want to hear! (See chapters 5 and 6 for more information on that very subject.)

But the core reason why people like dirty talk?

It's because all the areas of our brains are getting stimulated, usually at the same time as your body. Every cell in your brain is in use, and there can be a bit of overlap. Different sexual acts stimulate different areas in the brain, which decides which is likes and which it doesn't. The mind is our biggest sexual organ and one giant erogenous zone. The more stimulation it gets, the more the rest of your body is going to be running to catch up. Our brains are all about the feel-good chemicals like dopamine, the pleasure chemical, and oxytocin, the love hormone, and making your brain work harder actually helps increase these chemicals. The more you work to get them, the more you crave them, and the more you get.

There are even some psychologists who insist that an orgasm isn't just the arrival of a whole bunch of bodily fluids, it's actually a state of mind. Your goal is the orgasm, so as a result, you're thinking of the orgasm, and it makes it a hundred times better. A drawn-out, amazing, psychological phenomena. Cool, right?

The kind of sex you like, the foreplay you like, the people you're attracted to, this is all decided by your brain. Of course, your actual life affects what you like as well.

For example, it's a common theme in people who have a lot of power in their everyday life (think CEOs, politicians, and people in leadership roles) to enjoy more submissive-like sex, where they're at the mercy of someone else. They like being told how naughty they've been and how they're going to get punished. What kind of sex they want is an exact opposite thing of their everyday life.

But with all the good that comes with it, why does dirty talk feel so taboo and naughty? If we love it so much, why is it so awkward to think about doing or talk about?

Well, first off, let's get this out there: there is absolutely nothing wrong, dirty, or shameful about dirty talk. It can absolutely be an amazing and healthy addition to your sex life, and you'll enjoy yourself. Being open and knowing what you want is not a bad thing. Once you realize this and get more comfortable with it, it will get easier. But, you might not want to lose that feeling of "this is so naughty" because it can make it hotter, just saying.

Why do we see dirty talk as such a taboo thing? Well, it actually has to do with how we're raised. Despite the fact that sex is thrown at us at every corner, from advertisements to the magazines in the grocery store checkout lane to literally all over the internet (no, seriously, 30% of all data transferred across the internet is porn, and some porn sites get more streams more than Netflix and Hulu), sex is still regarded as something you just don't talk about. Yes, you may share some of your sexual escapades with your close friends, but for the most part, people keep their sex lives to themselves.

This starts in your childhood. You're told growing up that only 'bad kids' talk about sex, and you start to see sex as a shameful topic that should never be mentioned, much less actually spoken about. I doubt your parents actually had a decent conversation with you about sex (not that you want to, to be fair). Your first sexual adventures, whether they were porn, masturbation, or something else, were probably done in absolute secrecy, far away from any prying eyes. You've probably never even really talked about them to this day. It's ingrained in you that it's bad to talk about sex from a young age, and this affects us as we become adults.

We just have a hard time discussing it. Picture yourself walking up to your partner and telling them outright that you want to have sex right then, right now, right there. No warning. It makes you uncomfortable, right?

Some of the blame rests with the name. "Dirty talk". Like what's written above, dirty talk is not filthy, it's not gross, it's not bad. It's a way of you expressing yourself sexually, and that is never a bad thing. You're going to read that, over and over again, until you believe it. It's also going to show up a lot in the coming chapters.

But remember, dirty talk can be fun. It can be liberating. It can feel naughty and sexy and taboo and make you feel like a "bad boy/girl". It can make your sex life better, ignite your confidence, and there's so much variety to it, you're bound to find something that you like.

But, if you're still unsure on whether or not dirty talk makes things better, here are some reasons why you should give it a try;

1) Fewer communication problems. Better communication equals better sex. Dirty talk is all about telling your partner what you want to do, what they want to be done to them, and what feels good. Which means that if something is working, you'll know it. At the same time, if something is not working, you will know it. There is no downside.
2) Reignites the flame. People who have been dating for a long time can relate to this. When you've been at it for a while, the excitement and passion inevitably burn out. It's unfortunate, but it happens. It's natural and normal, and thankfully, it can be fixed with a little work and some variety. Dirty talk is a good way to fix this and break out of that sexy rut.
3) Stronger connection. If your communication in the bedroom improves, then your communication overall with your partner will improve. Doing something that could be potentially be embarrassing with someone who you love and trust will only make things better and bring you closer. It could even lead to potentially making it easier to talk about trying more things in the bedroom.
4) Inspires your sex life. Dirty talking can feel uncomfortable and awkward at first, but with time, and practice, and just

like any new thing, it gets better. You'll be more confident in trying more new, hotter things, like experimenting with toys or new positions.

5) It can be done anywhere. One of the huge benefits of dirty talk is that it is incredibly versatile and it is in no way just for the bedroom. There is really no place where it can't be done. Dirty talk can be whispering what you want to do to your partner as you walk past them in the kitchen, or it can be sending them a sexy text during the work day. There are no limits, as long as you're both into it!
6) Confidence. No, you read that right. Trying new things in your bedroom actually leads to more confidence in other parts of your life. If you can be open to trying something new in a defenseless and vulnerable place like the bedroom, you can do anything!

So, really, with all these reasons to try dirty talk, what's stopping you? Really, what's stopping you from making your sex life better, for you and whatever partner you may have?

Practice Makes Perfect

Things to remember as you go into the big, beautiful, and sexy world of dirty talk!

Relax. This is easier said than done. Relaxing can be difficult, especially when it's something you've never done before. Just take a deep breath and remember that the more you do this, the better and more relaxed you get.

Worry will kill your game. It will take practice, and you won't do it perfectly right away. Just keep trying, see what works and what does not. It will naturally get better over time.

It's OK to be nervous. Even if your partner has been doing this for years, they had their first time talking dirty. Be honest and tell your partner that you're feeling a bit anxious, and they'll likely understand.

You being comfortable is important. Don't do anything you're not comfortable with. If you're not completely comfortable at the idea of talking dirty, speak with your partner about it. If there is something that they can do, or you can do, to make you more comfortable with the idea, do it!

Communicate, communicate, communicate. There is never too much communication in a relationship, especially a sexual one where you're constantly put in a vulnerable and open place. Communication is essential to any fantastic, mind-blowing sex.

Be yourself. This goes along with not doing anything you're not 110% comfortable with. Say what you yourself would like to hear. It's pretty likely that it's similar to what your partner would want to hear.

Have fun. This is the most important step of all, because, really, if you're not having fun during sex, what exactly is the point of having sex? If talking dirty doesn't work for you, it's no big deal. If you're not having a good time, you don't have to do it. It's really that simple. The worst that could happen is you mess up and you and your partner have a good laugh before trying again. Don't worry and just have fun!

Do's and Don'ts!

It can be tricky to get the hang of dirty talk. But, worst comes to worst, you and your partner will have a funny story to tell.

Do Fake it Till You Make It. Even if you're a giant bundle of nerves with absolutely no idea what to say and would rather just not have sex instead of saying to your partner to "do it again", act confident. It's more about how you say it than what you're saying, believe it or not. So, even if you say something completely out of context, as long as you use the right tone of voice, you can make it sound hot.

Don't worry if you sound like you're just spouting cheese. Dirty talk is cheesy. That's just a fact. There are only so many ways you can say "I want to make you come," and on that list, there's probably only a few that will really get your partner going. Just keeping trying, and eventually, you'll find the perfect one. When talking dirty works, it really works.

Do be honest. If something is not working for you, tell them. Don't lie and say things are working when they're not. Keep in mind you should be telling them what is working for you. The key is keeping your partner updated.

Don't be negative. Don't tell your partner what they're doing wrong in a negative way. Make sure to emphasize what they're doing right rather than what they're doing wrong. Something like "I really like what you did there, do that again." Also, make sure the negatives about your own skills. Really focus on what you know you're good at or what feels right to say. And if you say something wrong, don't mull over it.

Do keep it simple. Even just simple phrases like "yes" and "right there" work like a charm. Like. A. Charm. Yes, it's a small step, but it's still a step. Keeping things light and easy is a perfect way to start off your dirty talking journey.

Don't just stay in your comfort zone. Comfort zones, or doing the same thing over and over again, can get old after a while. Your sex life is probably great the way it is, but there's nothing wrong with a little variety. The whole point of trying dirty talk, if you've never done it before, is to try and shake things up in your life. The first few times you try dirty talk, it may seem awkward and uncomfortable, but eventually, you'll have an entirely new kind of comfort zone.

What NOT to say

Before we go into what you should say, we're going to cover what you should not say.

The rules of what not to say during dirty talk are the same rules you use for Thanksgiving dinner; or any major holiday where there are family members present. Basically, if you think to yourself "this will start a fight and just doesn't have a place here", probably just don't say it. But just in case, here are some examples, and the best part, they're pretty standard, so you shouldn't have a hard time.

Keep in mind, if you're into any of these things, no judgment. You do you.

Politics: This should be a no-brainer, but just don't. Considering our recent political climate, and the tension in general, it just does not have a place in the bedroom. Especially, if you don't know your partner very well.

The To-Do List: The bedroom should be a place to get away from these things. It should be a no stress environment. You're supposed to be having fun, not thinking about whether or not you should do laundry or the next time you have to take out the garbage.

Fights you've had: The bedroom is not the place to suddenly start remembering a reason for why you're mad at them. That can wait. Don't be talking about how sexy they are and then just start bringing up an argument that you had in the past few weeks. The last thing you want is to start having an argument right in the middle of sex. It's not fun.

Family members: This may not be one that you don't talk about at Thanksgiving, but really. Your grandmother, your family drama, or the crazy thing your mom did last week does not belong anywhere near your sex life.

Just general unpleasant, not sexy things: This one really does not need an explanation. Anything that immediately makes you think "oh gross", just don't say it.

Basically, the main rule about what not to say during sexy talk is just using your common sense. Common sense exists for a reason. (The reason is to keep your dirty talk game up, obviously.)

When Things Go Wrong

Things go wrong. This is just a part of life. Yes, it happens in the bedroom, especially when you're trying something new. You've said the wrong things, or you've completely broken character and started laughing, or you're just completely blanking on what to say and stumbling over your words. Here's what you do.

1) BREATH. It's OK. It happens. It's totally fine. You are not the first person to screw up during dirty talk, and you will not be the last. You're a newbie at this, don't forget.
2) Remember, it's temporary. Yes, this may be utterly mortifying at this very moment, but pretty soon, this moment will be gone and just be a distant memory. Pinky promise.
3) It's all in how you react to it. OK, you can't control what has gone wrong, but you can control how you behave in the face of it. Your reflex may be to freak out and cry or just shut down or all of the above, don't. It will reflect much better on you if you're calm or try to laugh it off. Your reaction can say a lot about who you are. Remember, this is something you can control.

4) Look at your partner's reaction. Just like your reaction says a lot about you, it will say a lot about them. Their attitude about it will likely reflect yours. If you act awkward about it, they'll be awkward. If you laugh about it and brush it off, they will too. They might be specifically waiting for your reaction. And remember, if it's your first time, awkwardness sometimes just comes with the territory.
5) Accept it happened. You might find yourself going through the five stages of grief over this. Denial ("no way I said that, this is horrible and awkward, no way"), anger ("I'm an idiot, so embarrassed, this is stupid"), bargaining ("maybe they didn't hear, I'll give anything for them not to have heard that, all the gold in the world"), depression ("I am never trying dirty talk ever again, I am the worst ever") and acceptance ("okay, that happened, it's time to move on"). Accept it happened and you can move on. It's OK if it takes time before you want to try it again.
6) Don't take this as a sign that you shouldn't try again, and actually try again. The first time doing anything that you've never done before, or something you're not completely comfortable with, can be nerve-wracking. It will get better and easier. You wouldn't stop cooking just because you've burned your first casserole, would you? It takes practice, and sometimes just a little bit of direction. Go get 'em, you sexy beast, you!

When you are ready to try again, here's another piece of advice: Don't focus on the past, be in the present, and most importantly, have realistic expectations on yourself. Maybe, the reason you messed up is that you were in way over your head. You've never tried dirty talk before, but you decided to jump right into hardcore role play. Having expectations is fine, but make sure they're realistic. Identify the reason and try to deal with it.

Your first time trying to talk dirty may not go all that great. It's going to go far from perfect and you'll probably mess up the first time, or the first few times, you try it. You can't change that. When you do, try again and be positive. Think of all the things that are going to go right, rather than all the things that are going to go wrong. Don't worry too much about it. Look at the bright side, you'll just have a funny story you can tell later on.

If you're really feeling anxious about trying again, talk to your partner about it. Ask for help and get their opinion on it. If they're someone who's been talking dirty for a long time, they'll probably be able to make you feel better and tell you their own stories. They've probably messed up, too! If they're new to this as well, you two can work together to make it better.

Now, if it's your partner that says the wrong things, and not you, don't make a huge deal about it. Unless it's something that actually needs your attention right at that very moment, do your best to brush it off and move on. Your partner is not going to say all the right things all the time, and sometimes, they might say something you're not expecting. You might not know how to react, and you might even find yourself shocked, maybe even disgusted.

In the heat of the moment, people aren't usually going to say things that they would normally say. Dirty talk often generates pictures in your mind, and the farther you go and the hotter it gets, more and more images are flashing through your head, a lot of them a fantasy. The more a person gets with the idea of exploring their fantasies, they're going to start thinking of things that have never occurred to them before.

Imagine this: when you're really horny, is the thought of what sounds coming out of your mouth anywhere near the forefront of your brain? No, you're probably just lost in the heat and the passion of it all and the last thing you're thinking about what's coming out of your mouth or what's sprinting through your mind. You just want to get there.

It's the exact same with dirty talk. Your partner is not thinking about what they're saying when they're really in the heat of the moment. It's not a reflection on you; it's just all about what gets you going.

Types of Dirty Talk

Yes, there are kinds of dirty talk. But it basically falls into five simple categories.

Now, if all of this seems daunting, just remember this; before sex, say what you want. During sex, say what you like.

Present: This way is pretty simple and the easiest one to get the hang of. It doesn't require a lot of imagination. Think of it like being a narrator of the story of your sexual escapades, telling your story to someone else. Another way to think of it is being a sports commentator at a game. You can do it while you're, ahem, *doing it.*

Something like this: "Yeah, baby, right there. Mmm, you're so good. That feels so good. You taste amazing, babe. You're so hot. Do you like that? Oh, yeah, right there! I love how your skin feels under my hands. Your body's so sexy. You look so good right now. I'm kissing you. I want to f*** you right now. You like that, don't you?"

Tip: Lots of eye contact and be sincere. If something's not working, say so.

Future: This way requires a bit more of a thought process and some more imagination, but just think of it as what you plan on doing with the other person. Even if you just plan on doing missionary style, even just telling it to your partner that you definitely plan on doing it tonight or the next two minutes for that matter can really amp up the intensity. Really emphasize just how much you *want* it.

Try this: "I can't wait for tonight. I'm going to f*** you so hard. You look so hot in that and I can't wait to get it off you. When we get home, you better be naked."

Tip: Whisper it into your partner's ear in public. It will be the only thing on their mind until you two get alone and they can act on it.
Past: There is nothing wrong with a bit of reminiscing, especially the sexual kind. Doing it with your partner is even more fun. You can try to recreate the experience, and you might even have a better time the second time around.

Example: "Remember the time on Valentine's Day last year? Babe, you were so good. You looked so hot in that shirt. I loved licking that chocolate syrup off you. You felt amazing. We should do that again."
Tip: Surprise them! Just mention it and start talking.

Fantasy: Everyone fantasizes. Everyone has fantasies they visit again and again, and even if they're entirely unrealistic, they can get very spicy. This is not about telling your partner about your orgy fantasy (unless you know they're into that) but about getting them excited about your fantasy and their role in it.

Example: I had this dream the other night that you were the ruler of an island, and I was your war captive. You ordered me on my hands and knees and you spanked me until I was begging you to f*** me. You f***** me right from behind like an animal."

Tip: If you do go the dream direction, tell them in the morning when the two of you aren't rushing for work. Morning sex will wake you up faster than your morning coffee will!
Roleplay: Roleplay is when you act out a scenario using characters, and no, it's not just for hardcore BMSM. This is the hardest one and it can be daunting for beginners, so don't just jump into it right away. There is no end to the list of choices to make. Teacher-student, maid-master, doctor-nurse, a woman who can't pay for pizza-pizza boy, strangers at a bar. Another idea to try is picking a porn you both like and recreating it. It can get as kinky or as vanilla as you like, and there's nothing wrong with it. Just do what you're comfortable with, pick a safe word, and go with it.

Example: “I’m so sorry for not finishing my homework. I know I’ve been a bad boy/girl. Is there anything I can do?”
“There is something you can do.”
“Oh, thank you, I’ll do anything.”
“You’ve been bad, haven’t you?”

Tip: Recreate one of your own fantasies! Pick a fantasy that both you and your partner are into for your first try. You’ll both come into it excited to live out something you’ve both thought about.

Basic Dirty Talking Tips

Master the tone. Dirty talk really comes all down to the tone of how you say things. You could quote a five-dollar gas station romance novel with “heaving breasts” and “bulges in pants”, and if you’re using the right tone, it will come off sexy. Try implementing a soft, husky quality into your voice.

Pay attention to your voice. Don’t speak too fast or loud. Speaking fast can come off as nervous behavior. Speaking slowly, drawing out your voice and certain syllables can be really hot. Example: “Heeeeey, baby.”

Use good grammar. This should be a no-brainer, but seriously, just talk correctly. Use present tense during, past tense after, and future tense before. Don’t say “I want to be inside you so bad” when you’re already inside them. Don’t talk about how much you’re looking forward to having sex when you’ve just finished. It’ll just confuse and distract from the moment.

Body language matters. If you’re complimenting their abs or breasts but not touching them, or if you’re saying how much you want them but coming off as standoffish, this resonates with your partner. They’re paying attention to not just your voice, but how your body is reacting. Tip: Talk about the part of their body as you run your hands over it. After telling them how much you want them, follow that up with a kiss.

Remember the details. Especially if you’re complimenting someone. Pay attention to the details of the other person. You don’t have to write poetry about them; even mentioning how hot you find someone’s eyes when they’re doing oral on you works.

Use all five of your senses. Touch, sound, taste, smell, and sight. Use these five basic senses to your advantage; they’re there for you to use. Mention the softness of lips, how good your partner smells and tastes.

Check with your partner on profanity beforehand. Some people like it, some don’t. It really depends. That’s why it’s so important to talk this over with your partner and communicate. If you can, actually discuss which words work on you and which words don't if you can't, the only real place to test this out is in the bedroom.

Push yourself (to a point): The whole point of trying dirty talking is that you push your comfort zone a little. While yes, it's important that you're comfortable and you enjoy yourself, it's also important that you try new things and you're not just doing the same old, same old, because it will get boring, not just for you, but for your partner as well.

Try texting first: Refer to the chapter on sexting for more information. Sexting is a great alternative if you're really nervous. It's a good way to dip your toe into the water. Text your partner while they're at work so you know they're thinking of you.

What to Say

Unfortunately, there is no one line, word, or saying that will get every person in the world going. The reality is, you don't know what your partner will like without you explicitly asking them or them volunteering the information. There is such a variety of things you can say and so many different ways to say them.

The kind of dirty talk your partner will like really all depends on them. They could be into really softcore stuff, or they're a seasoned veteran who wants to hear the dirtiest things you can think of. What's important to remember is to make sure your words are tailored to the person and the situation.

Don't forget that it's not just about saying the words. It's also about the moans, your body language, the sounds, and the movements. The whole point of dirty talk is to show them how much you're into them and how much you're enjoying yourself. If it doesn't come off as genuine, well, you're screwed (no pun intended).

Basic Easy Lines to Get You Started

There is no harm in trying something new, and definitely no harm in trying some basics at first. Basics work because they're the bedrock of any future activities you will partake in the future. Read on, then get down!

- "I want you." Quick. Simple. To the point. It's an easy way to proclaim your desire, and will always come off as genuine. You're also puffing up their ego, reminding them just how hot you find them.
- "You smell delicious." This one can be tailored to fit any of the five senses. But talking about how good they smell might alleviate any concerns they have about their body odors. This statement also shows that you're paying attention to them,

that you're in the moment, and making them feel more confident. It validates them and makes them feel special.

- "I love it when you _______." Draw their attention to the one thing they do really, really well. Something you enjoy, and if they know you enjoy it, they'll enjoy doing it to you.
- "I want to feel you _____." By giving them exact directions, you're making them feel more confident because they know you'll enjoy what they're about to do. It points them in the right direction. This is an especially effective way to make sure you're always getting what you want as well.
- "I want you naked, right now." Taking command of a situation is hot. It's sexy. The anticipation for them increases too. They'll wonder what you have planned and how it's going to play out. When will it start? What do you have planned? How will you do it?
- "What do you feel like doing to me right now?" Questions are a great way to start off, especially for beginners who are still figuring out exactly what to say. It takes the heat off you and puts the ball into your partner's court.
- "You're so naughty. I love it." Validation for your partner is never a bad thing. It tells them you like what they're doing, to continue, and that you're grateful.
- "I can't wait to feel you inside me."
- "I am so ready for you."
- "I want to ______."

Chapter 2: Some More Basics

When to Start

The great thing about dirty talk is how versatile it is. You can text your partner while on transit, you can whisper into their ear at a party filled with 20 of your closest relatives, or scream "yes! yes! yes!" as they're doing exactly what needs to be done to get you off.

There is no wrong time to start dirty talking, but the general rule is; the more buildup, the bigger the payoff.

It's like this; you really want a piece of cake. So, you spend the entire day wanting a piece of cake. You eventually get home and finally have the piece of cake, thinking to yourself the whole time, this piece of cake is so good. It's delicious. So moist, it practically melts in my mouth. That piece of cake probably tastes so much better than it does with you waiting for it and thinking about it than it would if you just decided to have a piece of cake randomly.

Even starting in the morning, telling your partner how hot they are and continuously reminding them just how sexy you find them throughout the day builds up over the day. By the time you're both home and in the same room, you'll be able to actually do something you've been thinking and planning all day. Both of your imaginations have been running wild all day, so you're both just ready to go.

Just think of it as a really long kind of foreplay. But it pays off, in huge ways and better orgasms.

Let's face it. That's all you really want in life.

Words Matter: Vocabulary Lesson

Words do matter. You may have read earlier that you could probably make the weirdest thing sound sexy in just the right tone, but there's a limit to how much that works.

It's also important that you like what you're saying and you're comfortable with it. Dirty talk isn't just about turning your partner on; it's also about turning you on. Just as a little exercise, try writing down some of the words that get you going, whether they're nouns, verbs, or adjectives. In this way, you start to develop your own style and way of talking dirty that is 100% yours.

Here's a few to get you started:

Nouns

Cock

D***

P****

Thighs

Tits

Nipple

Chest

Breasts

Boobs

Verbs

Spank

F***

Suck

Lick

Spread

Feel

Stroke

Bite

Adjectives

Hard

Nasty

Soft

Bad

Hot

Sexy

Good

Sweet

Yummy

Take these words and write them down (see chapter 9 for more about this). Figure out what words you like. Say them out loud. Use them. Write down some phrases, too, if you feel that would help.

Inspiration

While there are a lot of great phrases in this book, it never hurts to check out somewhere else for ideas. Just like an artist is constantly looking for the motivation behind their next great piece, you should never stop looking for things that you want to try in the bedroom.

One of the easiest ways to find inspiration is through porn. Porn has done a lot of bad things for sex, such as creating extremely unrealistic expectations for both men and women, it's also done a lot of good. Porn stars are professional at talking dirty. There is even an entire genre of porn dedicated to it. They might use words you've never even thought of. It can also be very cliché, corny, and funny. Some of the things these actors and actresses will say might just have you rolling on the floor. Laugh, but don't think there's not something worth looking into there. Study them anyway.

Some of dirty talking porn might feel a little bit over the top and intense for beginners. Somewhere, you might find a few hardcore ideas. Just a simple type into your favorite search engine will bring up hundreds of thousands of results, and you'll definitely find something that you like. You can find easy to say, not too hardcore phrases for the gentlest of lovemaking and hardcore, super-raunchy comments for when you're going at it hard enough to break the bed. Or when you're ready for that, whichever.

Another place to check out, if you're not into porn, is just plain old regular movies and TV shows. Think Secretary, or Mr. and Mrs. Smith, films with super hot sex scenes. You might get some creative roleplaying ideas too. And because films are actually specifically written to sound realistic and actually have to convince the audience that it could actually happen, you'll get ideas that feel more natural to say.

Don't forget to talk to your friends too. Yes, this may seem weird at first, but talking about your sex life with your friends can be really fun and a great bonding experience. You also might get some ideas. This is especially good if some of your friends have more experience in things than you do. Literally, everyone on planet earth has one of these things that is not afraid to try everything and has probably actually tried everything. Warning: You could find out more than you ever wanted to know. If your friends are willing to open up, take advantage of it.

Music. Music is full of sexy phrases and mantras. Music is all about the way it makes you feel and can be incredibly sexy. Some people even have sex song playlists, believe it or not. Music is also a great way to really get into your body and just lose yourself, something you should be doing during sex. A quick internet search can have a lot of potential for some super hot lyrics.

Another good place to look, if a bit unconventional, is asking phone sex operations. Yes, they still exist, and yes, they have probably heard it all. I doubt they would mind if you called and asked for tips if you really wanted to. Some of them have probably had another person call them, and they might just appreciate the downtime! The companies really don't care as long as they're keeping a client on the line. And it definitely will not be the most shocking or unusual request they've ever had.

Of course, as time goes on and you become more comfortable with the idea of dirty talk, ideas will start to come to you naturally. Actively working to be creative will always lead to more creativity. You'll start to think of naughty ideas and dirty thoughts that might even shock you a little.

Setting the Mood

Setting the mood is important for dirty talk.

Tidy up your room and pick up your underwear off the floor. Wash the sheets and make sure everything smells clean. Clean up your room if you know that's where the two of you are going to be doing it. Take a shower. Wear clean underwear. Make sure you feel good and comfortable before you try something you haven't done before. Put the necessities of everything you'll need in a basket by your bed, like lube, condoms, props like vibrators (if you use them), and really anything else you want to use or feel you need.

If you really want to go for it, try changing the lighting in your bedroom with some red or white Christmas lights. It will make the light in your bedroom soft and sexy. Candles are also a great option. You could also invest in something new to wear, like lingerie. Sprinkle your cologne or perfume all over the room. Do it for a couple of hours before you start, so your partner doesn't get knocked over by the smell. Put together a playlist of music that gets you in the mood.

It's not just the bedroom that might need some attention. When things go more hardcore, you might want to explore the rest of your place. Think, the kitchen, the shower, the couch in the living room, take your pick. Will you need some extra pillows on the couch? Is the shower dirty? Do you have some delicious things in the fridge for licking off your partner's body later?

All these details really just help you relax. It gives you less to worry about when the time actually comes. The idea is to make sure that all you're thinking about is the dirty talk, meaning you can completely immerse yourself in the moment and be able to use your mouth to its fullest potential.

Easing into It

If you've never done dirty talk before, it can be helpful to just ease into it gently. Doing something you've never done before, especially something so intimate, can be daunting and uncomfortable.

This is also for your partner's benefit. If you just immediately jump into it, it might be more of a turn off than a turn on, especially if they haven't done it before either. I mean, think about it, how would you feel if they just suddenly decided to talk about spanking you? You'll likely find yourself very confused and wondering what exactly is going through their head.

That's why it's important to gently ease yourself and your partner into the idea.

You need to get to a point where you're comfortable talking about sex with your partner. Ways to this can include mentioning to them an article you read about dirty talk or any other thing you want to try in the bedroom. When you see a sex scene that you find hot in a movie or on a TV show, mention how hot you find it. Leave a book or a magazine somewhere where you know they'll find it, bookmarked on the page you want them to read. Remind them how hot you find them as they're heading out the door. Get them a sexy gift, like lingerie or whipped cream and cherries. They will get the message.

There are a whole variety of ways to bring the conversation up with your partner and make it easier to speak about with them. Doing this will make it easier for when you actually do start to do the deed. It's also a very sexy, subtle way that lets your partner know that you are thinking about your sex life and you find them desirable.

When you actually start getting down and dirty, start off with something familiar. Something you've thought in your head. Find things you love about their body, like their ass, their shoulders, their breasts, their naughty bits, take your pick. Compliment them. This should be easy because likely you've already had a lot of good thoughts about your partner's body. Just voice them.

Ask them questions. Tell them to talk to you. Ask them things like what would they like to do and where. Give them directions if you're feeling up for it. Use a lot of adjectives like "hot" or "wet". Remind them how sexy they are.

Making it easy for you and your partner, at least when you're starting out, is very important. Of course, that's why you picked up this book, so you're on the right track!

More Easy Lines

Just to get you more into it, here are some lines to help you:

- "Tell me what you want me to do to you. Right now." This line works especially well if you're running a bit of a blank or you're feeling a bit unsure about what they like.
- "Don't stop. Keep going. Right there." Simple. Easy. To the point.

- "I wish there weren't so many people around. If they weren't here, you'd be in for a surprise." Whisper this into your partner's ear somewhere in public.
- "I'm so turned on right now." If your partner does something especially sexy that comes out of nowhere, this is not a bad thing to say.
- "You're so sexy when you do that. Do it again."
- "That feels incredible. Please don't stop." Yes, this phrase comes off as tame, but it provides validation, and by saying please, you're putting them in control.
- "Just like that." Encouragement is never a bad thing. You should always tell your partner when they're doing something right.
- "I can't think of anything hotter than your face when you come." There are a lot of people out there who feel a bit insecure about how they look when they come. This will help them get more comfortable. It will always tell them that you enjoy bringing them pleasure so you can see that face again.
- "The sounds you make drive me crazy." This line is great to use on a partner who might be really quiet. There is a good possibility they're just insecure about how they sound.
- "Let's see how many times I can make you come." This ups the fantasy, as your partner immediately starts to picture the

very act and starts to guess the number. They'll start thinking of all the things you can do and will do to make it happen.

Chapter 3: It's Not You, It's the Talk

So, you (or your partner) isn't into it. Don't worry, it's totally normal, and there's probably a good reason for it.

Ultimately, whether or not someone like dirty talk is really just a matter of taste. It's not a reflection on you or your partner, and it's totally and completely normal. You're never going to be able to find a partner with whom you share all your sexual tastes with, and if you claim you have, one of you is a liar. It's like expecting to find someone who likes and dislikes all the same foods as you.

Well, some people like broccoli and some people don't. You might like chicken parmesan and maybe your partner is a vegetarian. No two people have the exact same palate, just as no two people have the exact same sexual needs and wants. You'll find people with similarities, but you won't find a perfect match. And that's OK. All it means is it's not your thing. But, you might be with a person who does like it.

As long as you and your partner communicate, you'll do fine. With that in mind, here are a few reasons why it's totally normal and valid to dislike dirty talk because no, your partner is not a freak.

Why It's Totally Fine (And Normal) to Not Like Dirty Talk

1) You don't need the play by play. Present dirty talk (the act of narrating your actions as you are doing them) can often be a little bit like a bad sports' commentator. Unnecessary, irritating, and sometimes, you just want to be there for all the actions. You don't need someone telling you what they're doing; you can see and feel it, so why?
2) You've never even tried it. You think it's kind of ridiculous, and you're just not into even trying it. That's OK. Just remember this: dirty talk is a lot of different things, and might not be what you're thinking of. If the issue is insecurity-based, think of it as a food you've never tried before. How do you know you don't like it if you have never tried it before?
3) Porn. Porn, while great in a lot of ways, has unfortunately created very unrealistic views of what sex is, and dirty talk is only one part of that. In porn, dirty talk is basically just a man saying "yeah, you want that" or "you've been a bad girl" while the woman goes "yeah yeah yeah". Yeah, no.

Porn dirty talk, when translated to real life sex dirty talk, seems rehearsed, forced, and feigned. And it is kind of hilarious.

4) It's a quickie. Sometimes, people just want to get in and get out. Dirty talk has a tendency to draw out the experience, and the other person just wants to get a move on. Wham, bam, thank you, Mam. They just want to get back to their lives, whether it's work or parenting or whatever else they have going on in their lives.
5) It can feel forced. Dirty talk can seem disingenuous and, well, forced if not done naturally. When it's blindingly obvious that a partner is just doing it because you like it or because "that's what you do during sex", not because they're into it, it can be a real turn off. Really, try to only talk dirty if that's how you're actually feeling.
6) Less talking, more doing. People talk all day. It's just part of our society and what we do. They talk to their coworkers, their friends, their family, you, so maybe when they get to the dirty, they just don't want to. Silence and sex are not necessarily a bad mixture.
7) It's a distraction. Some people find it difficult talking dirty during sex because they find it takes the focus away from the actual sex. They're sidetracked by the talking and have a hard time getting their focus on what's actually going on. Of course, do keep in mind that for some people, they have the

opposite problem. They need the talk to keep their mind focused on the task.

8) You think of dirty talking as only "one thing". Some people really only consider dirty talking as, well, talking while doing the dirty. It's a lot of other things other than that, including sexting, role play, games, and sharing fantasies. Maybe you should try some of these.
9) Your partner (or you) is just not that great at it. Look, we all have things we are good at. Some people are good at cooking, others are good at writing, and for others, maybe it's dirty talking. But not everybody has this talent, and *that's okay*. This doesn't mean there isn't room for improvement and you can get better at using your mouth in an entirely different way. Finding a partner with whom you can explore and try new things with is a dream.
10) You like what you like, and that's all there is to it. You do not have to explain your sexual wants, needs, likes, or dislikes to anyone. Some people like dirty talk and some people don't. That's really all there is to it. There is nothing wrong with you, and it's completely and totally natural.

What to Do If You Don't Like Dirty Talk (And Your Partner Does)

One thing that happens when you've been in a relationship for a long time is that the passion and the lust that were so big at the start of your relationship start to fade out. This will, if you want it to, lead to the two of you exploring your sexual likes and dislikes together, hopefully trying new things.

This part of your relationship can be really fun and exciting. You learn about each other and open yourself up to the other person in ways you might not have done before. You might learn about things that you've never even thought to try, and you really like them. The entire Kama Sutra is your oyster. The more you talk about sex and explore sex, the better your sex life and your relationship will be.

Dirty talk could be one of these things you can try. But it doesn't work for everyone. Maybe it doesn't work for you. But it really works for your partner. Maybe, your reasons are listed above, or maybe it's an entirely different one. It doesn't really matter. What matters is that you're both having a good time. Remember, your partner wants you to enjoy yourself. They want you to come away from the encounter pleased. Here are some things you can try:

1) Try a different kind of dirty talk. Maybe it's not the dirty talk that's not doing it for you; maybe it's the kind of it. Maybe you're really into present dirty talk, but try role play. Maybe try a fantasy. There are no limits.
2) Change the environment. Maybe, you're really not into the idea of whispering in your partner's ear in a public place, but maybe they are. Changing an aspect of the environment you're in can help.
3) Be genuine. Maybe, you're just not into it because it's coming off as fake or impersonal. If that's something that matters to you, this may be it. If all your partner is saying "your body is so hot", well, that's pretty vague. Ask them to be a bit more personal. Tell them to be more specific.
4) Stretch your comfort zone. One of the biggest reasons people don't want to try dirty talk is because they're not comfortable with it. Well, the only way to get comfortable with something is to do it over and over again.
5) Try something else. In the end, if dirty talk doesn't work for you, it doesn't work for you. It's no big deal and think of this as a "one door closes, another door opens" kind of deal. Onward to the next sexual adventure!

If You Really Like It (But Your Partner Does Not)

Of course, the exact opposite situation might happen to you. You might really like dirty talk, but maybe your partner hates it, for whatever reason.

Here's what you can do about it.

First: No, your partner is not a freak. Something is not wrong with them. They just have different sexual wants than you have. They just get turned on by different things. That's really all there is to it. You need to approach this, and really, any other sexual request they have in the future, with an open-minded attitude.

Second: Find out why they don't like dirty talk. Maybe, it's because it seems very forced. Maybe, they just don't want to talk during sex. Maybe, they're into something completely different. For all you know, maybe they haven't even tried it. Whatever it is, they will probably have a reason.

Third: Try a different kind of dirty talk. Maybe, they just want to try something else. Dirty talk can be switched up all the time, so don't worry about them not liking dirty talk. Experiment a little!

Fourth: Try new things and find something that works for both of you. Sex should be fun for both of you, so hopefully, by working together and communicating, you'll get there.

If Your Partner Just Has Never Tried It Before

Having a partner that has done something that you haven't can be a bit daunting. It's like having sex with someone for the first time and you've already done it. You want their expectations to be met because it's their first time. On top of that, the person who has never had sex before is probably worrying about whoever came before them, and whether or not they'd compare.

Dirty talk is the same way. If you've done it a lot but your partner has never done it, this could be stressful on them. They could be feeling a bit insecure and awkward about it. They're also very likely curious about it, as most people are when they come across something they haven't tried before. You can use this.

First: Try to get into your partner's head and try to help them get into yours. Explain to them why you like it. Let them know why it's great. Try to get them curious and wondering. People are naturally curious creatures. Yes, curiosity killed the cat, but it hasn't stopped people from continuing to explore things that they don't understand or they're not familiar with.

Second: Let them know what they're doing good. Make sure they know how great they are at doing that one thing that gets you going. Make them feel sexy. If you want your partner to do sexy things, they need to feel sexy. Compliments get you far, making them feel more confident and empowered. You really don't want them to start thinking you need something more.

Third: Make sure they're comfortable with the idea. The last thing you want is to corner your partner into something they're just not into trying. Don't guilt them into it. Don't make it sound as if you absolutely need it. If they're not at least willing to give it a try, it's just going to be bad.

Fourth: Take it slow. Don't expect them to get it absolutely perfect on the first try. They're probably going to be nervous and will trip over their tongues a bit. They need to get used to doing it first. One step at a time. Remember your first time trying dirty talk? They probably feel just as awkward and out of place as you did.

Fifth: Be specific. Telling someone "I want you to talk dirty to me" can come off as very vague, especially if they haven't done it before. They may have no idea where to begin. If you've already done it, you probably already know what you like and what you like said to you. Give them a keyword or tell them a line you like to hear. Have requests and ask questions, such as "you like that, baby?" or "tell me how much that turns you on". Make suggestions. And when they run with it, let them. Buy them this book. It's helping you, right?

Sixth: Level the playing field. Tell them about your first experience dirty talking and how it went. You might even have some funny stories to break the tension and make them feel more confident. They might have some funny stories about their own sexual experiences that went wrong. Something about another person who you want to have sex with opening up about their own funny moments can definitely make you hotter.

Seventh: No means no. Always. At the end of the day, if you can't convince someone to try something, just take their answer as final. If they say no, you have to either evaluate the relationship (if dirty talking is really that important to you), or you have to just accept their answer. Consent matters.

If Your Partner Is Really Just Not Good at It

This is the worse. You're really into dirty talk, you know you're into hearing how hot you are when your orgasm, and … your partner is terrible at it. Some people are just not good at dirty talk. It happens. Some people are naturally good at it, while others aren't. It's nothing that can't be fixed, thankfully.

Why Your Partner Might Be Bad at It

1) They've never done it before. They might be a complete newbie at the whole dirty talk game. For all you know, you could've been the first person to even ask it of them.
2) They're nervous. Maybe they've done dirty talk before, but they're just unable to relax. They feel awkward and are treating the whole experience like they're going to war.
3) They just don't know what to say. They might just not be the wordy type.
4) They don't like dirty talk. It goes both ways. If your partner is not into dirty talk, it's likely that they won't enjoy doing it. If they're genuinely trying, you should give them some points for that, but if they're being a brat, well, who wants that?

So, the question is, do you tell them? The answer to that will always be yes. Even if it's a one-night stand and you never plan on seeing them again, you should still let them know that dirty talk is not one of their strong suits or if something just isn't working. All you're doing is making it worse for you and making the next person deal with it.

Of course, you don't want to hurt or embarrass your partner. You don't want them to just never want to try it again because what if you really like it and need it to get it off? It will just be another uphill battle to come out and say "you're bad at this." At the same time, you don't want to be hearing awkward, cringe-worthy, not-so-hot nothings whispered in your ear for the rest of your life.

Thankfully, there are some things you can do.

1) Tell them what you like. If you like being told that you have an amazing ass, tell them. Really communicate what you want. Having an open conversation can be really helpful; for all you know, they have some things that you do that they don't particularly like.
2) Compliment them. Make sure you let them know when they're doing something right. At the same time, if they're doing something wrong, gently guide them in the right direction. Make suggestions as to what they can try.
3) Try not to hurt their feelings. Try to avoid just coming out and saying that they're bad at dirty talk. Instead, focus on what their strengths. Negativity is really not the answer here and might just cause from friction. Not the good kind.
4) Encourage them by talking dirty to them. They might just need to get some of the creative juices flowing. An easy way to do this is to talk dirty to them; they might follow your lead.

When all else fails, well, this is what this book is for, right?

And if that still doesn't work, you might actually have to address the problem. Sit down with them and say: "you're not great at this. I'm sorry. Can we talk about this?" You might hurt their feelings, but it's really better in the long run.

Dirty Talk That Isn't Dirty Talk

Just because there are voices involved doesn't necessarily constitute as dirty talk, but it can still have the same effect. If you're one of these people who don't, but your partner really likes it, or vice versa, you might find something you want to try here.

1) Read erotica to each other. There are plenty of websites online with free erotica that you can read to the other, or I'm sure that one of you has a favorite dirty story somewhere. Take it to bed with you, and maybe do a bit of kinky foreplay to up the sexiness.
2) Moan instead. Dirty talk just may be your partner's way of knowing that you're having a good time. Maybe they just need to hear you say something like "that's so good". Try moaning; it has the same effect, but you don't actually need to speak. If they're doing something right, it should come

naturally. Moaning is also a great step if you want to talk dirty but you're not quite comfortable with it yet.

3) Speak in another language. This one can be a little iffy, especially if you're one of these people who just don't want to talk during sex. But there are people out there who find foreigners sexy just for having a slight accent. Also, knowing another language is scientifically proven to make you smarter, so if your partner is really into intelligence, this may work for you. Speaking another language during sex is different. Even just a few sexy phrases could help. Think French, the language of love. *Voulez vous coucher avec moi ce soir?*
4) Play some sex games. Check out the role play chapter for a whole host of games you can play with your partner. Everything from role play to sexy word games, there's no limit to what you can try. These can be great if your partner is just not wordy, or is not comfortable talking about sex.
5) Use your pen. Whip out a pen and some paper, and write a note to your partner, including how sexy they look and all the hot things you want to do to them. Check out the pen and paper section of sexting for more ideas!
6) Music. Music is a great way to communicate with your partner. Remember when everyone was dedicating songs to their partners on the radio? There was a good reason. There's nothing like getting a song sent to you and your partner

making a point to say it reminds you of them. Tip: Beyoncé is a good place to start.

The reality is, at the end of the day, you might just not be sexually compatible. It's up to you as to how you want to go forward if you realize this. There's nothing wrong with you, and there's nothing wrong with them. You just want different things in the bedroom. Maybe, this will mean that you will end it right there and then, but maybe, it won't be too much of an issue. But once you figure that out, you can move forward.

Chapter 4: The Power of Your Pen (and Your Keyboard)

Dirty talk is not just face-to-face. Dirty talk is also in other ways of communication. In the world of social media, phone lines, and the mailman, it's popularity is still very much alive and pumping.

And don't think it's not just for long distant couples. It can be fun for couples who live in the same area. For couples who see each other every day, it's a great way to make yourself more excited to see each other. Send your partner a text during the day about how much you want to see them in what they're wearing right now. Give them a call to remind them of the hot sex you had that very morning. Write a note in the mirror, as they are showering, about how much you wished you could be in there with them.

There's no harm in it, and it can be fun coming up with creative ways to surprise your partner. Especially when they're not expecting it.

Sexting

Once upon a time, in an entirely different world, phone sex used to mean whispering over the phone to your partner. While this is still actually extremely hot, and absolutely a viable option, phone sex is now all about the sexting; sex over text. It's definitely not limited to just texting, either. You can do it on messenger and dating apps too.

This can be anything from a super sexy picture to a flirty message. There are very few limits to what sexting actually is. Sexting is great because it can be many different things. It can be foreplay for what's to come later, or it can actually be the main event if you're in a long distant relationship.

What was started by teenagers trying to hide their sex lives from their parents has turned into something that nearly every person with a smartphone has indulged in at one point or another. It's fun, it's easy, and considering that there's no such thing as a smartphone without a camera anymore, extremely popular.

The basic, cardinal rules to sexting:

1) If you're going to send pictures, make sure you're unidentifiable in them. This is an important rule to follow. The last thing you want is for your pictures to end up online, or being used as blackmail. This is actually a very common problem with real legal consequences, so think really hard.

2) Also, if you're going to send pictures, make sure the background is good. Your partner does not need to see your pile of dirty laundry in the corner!
3) Use emojis. Which ones you use are totally up to you, but they really add some personality into your messages. Winky faces are equal parts cute and sexy!
4) Make sure the other person is interested. And don't shame the other person if they're not!
5) Use good grammar. This tip is wholly underrated. "Sup" is definitely less sexy than "hey, cutie, what are you up to?"
6) Keep your responses coming quick. Nothing ruins the mood faster during sexting than someone who waits an hour to text back. You really just don't want to go there.
7) Be appropriate. When you sext is important. Don't be that person who sends them a naked picture when they're in the middle of a meeting at work. Be sure that they're alone, or, if they're not alone, they're in a place where they can get alone quickly.
8) Keep it simple, and start slow. Jumping right into the sex talk is fine, but it can come off as thirsty. A simple "Hey, hottie, I've been thinking about you :)" goes a long way.
9) Nix the emotions. Sexting is really not a romantic thing. Don't bring that into it.
10) Stretching the truth is fine. Sexting is really just about the fantasy. It's fun.

11) Don't be afraid to use sexting as a way to coach your partner, or talk about fantasies. Sexting is great because you can often describe situations that you want to happen in real life. Most people will take the hint if you say specifically "I love it when you do that" or "you should do that more often."
12) Remember that sexting does not automatically mean sex. Just because a person spent the whole day sending you sexy messages is not an invitation to actually go over and have sex. Make sure you have their explicit consent.

How to Sext

1) Start off subtly. Something like saying hello. Just catch their attention, and make sure they can give you 100% of theirs.
2) Keep it classy (at first). Don't jump right into the sex talk. It can come off as trashy and gross. It might even turn them off. Ask them how their day is going, what they have planned for the rest of the day, whether or not they're busy.
3) Compliment them. Refer to the last time you saw them, like a picture on their online dating profile. Compliments work to get the mood going.
4) If you're running dry on creativity, ask them "What would you like to do to me?"

Examples (And Why They Work)

What's your fantasy?

Why it works: This one is great because you learn and get an idea for future romps. Other questions like "what would you do with me right now" and "do you ever think of me in that way?" are also perfect.

Your _____ feels incredible.

Why it works: Compliments that actually feel genuine are always better than compliments that just seem thrown out there. Your partner wants to know what you like about them and what they're good at, whether it be their tongue, fingers, lips, etc.

You looked so hot in ____. I want to see you wear it again.

Why it works: This can be a subtle way to work pictures into the game, or actually get the two of you making plans for seeing each other in person. You could also follow it up with an "I bet it looks so much better on the floor" if you're feeling really bold.

Come under the blankets and warm me up.

Why it works: Subtly telling your partner you definitely want to heat things up always is the way to go. This is a great one for just starting off.

I can't wait for you to come...home.

Why it works: This comes off as sexy, playful, and shows you've got a sense of humor. Extra points for incorporating a pun. This one is great if your partner is just leaving work or away from you for a while.

You're all mine tonight.

Why it works: Reminding your partner how much you want them is never a bad thing. Knowing that you're looking forward to seeing them and you find them hot will make them think about you all day.

What are you wearing?

Why it works: It's easy, it's a great way to break the ice into sexting, and it's a good opening for the other person to send a picture.

Before you try with an actual partner, you could log onto an online sex chat site (yes, they exist) and try out some lines there. See the reactions on the site and really test out what works and what doesn't. You can try out new messages you've thought of, find other ideas, and best of all, the anonymous nature of it means that if you do mess up, nobody will ever know. Well, nobody important, anyway.

You can really put your thoughts and feelings out there without worrying too much. After all, why do you care? It's not like you're ever going to meet these people in real life. If you say something that shocks or repulses them, they'll just tell you and you can move on. They don't know you, so they can be honest with you without worry.

Phone Sex: It Doesn't Belong in The Past

Don't leave this one in the dark ages! Phone sex is still alive and well. Phone sex operators are very popular around the world. It's not going anywhere for a long, long time, and it shouldn't go anywhere, *ever*.

Phone sex has been around since phones were invented. Of course, phone lines used to be called "party lines" where several people could listen to at once, so it probably wasn't quite as popular then. It would make for some awkward neighborhood gatherings. But someone, a genius whose name will never be known, took a shot, and phone sex was born.

That must have been a really hot session. Think about it; the thrill of getting caught plus all the sexiness equals some pretty good times. Phone sex really took off in the eighties, when phone sex operators became a thing. All it took was a phone and a credit card, and you were in. As time went on, it became easier and easier to participate, fast forwarding to today where our phones are tiny computers we carry around in our pockets.

While it used to be something that was a lot more shameful, now it's more accepted in society. It's used in long distance relationships to keep it alive and is actually expected. How else are you supposed to get hot and heavy with your partner when they're a hundred miles away? Phone sex or video chat sex is a great way to add some spice to your relationship, even if you're not in different cities. Go for it and try it: It's a lot of fun!

Like dirty talking, it can be a little awkward and uncomfortable at first, but with these tips, you'll be a master in no time!

1) Make sure that you're in a private area and you're comfortable. Especially, your first time trying it with a new partner. This can really be anywhere, wearing anything. It's

probably not a bad idea to wear something sexy to get you in the mood.

2) It's OK to lie. You're probably not wearing your sexiest lingerie, lounging around reading a magazine and you're probably not just about to get into the shower from a sweaty workout. That's OK. Phone sex, like sexting, is about the fantasy.
3) Know your partner. Phone sex is not all about actual phone sex. You can discuss non-sexual topics as well, like families, careers, and dating lives. Getting them to open up about themselves makes them more comfortable. The more comfortable they are, the more likely they will be to get into it.
4) Pay attention. You've probably seen these advertisements for sex phone operators where it shows a woman walking around her house doing laundry and cleaning their kitchen while moaning "yeah baby!" into her headset. This isn't at all accurate. Give 100% of your attention. Your partner will know if you aren't.
5) Engage. Ask them to clarify. Build on their fantasies. Be consistent.
6) Be open-minded. Society today is still judgmental towards certain kinks and fantasies, and your partner might be scared to know what you think, or embarrassed. Make sure your partner knows that you're open to trying new things and

want them to have a good time. Be open about it. You might actually enjoy it.

7) Don't rush. Be a bit of a tease. Describe every movement and take your time doing so. Delay and build up the pressure. It will drive them wild.
8) Reality doesn't matter. With phone sex, literally, everything is happening in your imagination. There are no limits. Want to have sex in the Eiffel Tower at midnight? Go for it. Want to have a threesome with Zeus and Hera in their palace in the sky with thunderbolts raining down on you? The choice is yours. Create characters. Add dimensions. Be people who you are definitely not. There. Are. No. Limits. Remember this, and you'll have an even better time.
9) Actually, move. Really get into the fantasy. If they say they're kissing you in the fantasy, squirm and move as if you were kissing them in real life.
10) Mix it up a bit, and really use your words. Make sure that you use the vocabulary your partner is comfortable with, but try to use different words. Description is literally everything during phone sex. Where are you sitting? What are you wearing? Use details and mix it up a bit. Don't just keep saying the same thing over and over again. It will help paint them a picture of the fantasy.

11) Use toys. If you're bored with just using your fingers, toys are a great alternative. Tell your partner you have it and let them direct you.
12) Use it to motivate your actual sex life. If you plan on meeting up with this person, try discussing things you actually want to do and try to remember specifically what your partner mentions. Talk about what you want your partner to wear and do. Try to remember if they make any requests. When you do it, they'll remember the call and the anticipation will drive them wild.

If you're really blanking, having a list of phrases, or even a template, in front of you isn't a bad idea. You don't even have to memorize some phrases, you can just write them down right in front of you. Sex phone operators actually use this very method when they're running out of things to say. You may feel dumb or stupid needing to refer to a cheat sheet, but take just a moment; it doesn't really matter as long as your partner doesn't actually know. Think of it as if you were a swimmer and you were using the edge of the swimming pool to kick off of. It won't get you all the way there, but having it will definitely help get you going.

Templates and Phrases to Try

I love how your _____ feels when you do _____.

I want to do ____ again.

Tell me what you want to do to me.

I want to feel you ____.

Of course, if you're really struggling with it, there's always the option of calling up an actual phone sex operator and asking them if they have any ideas. You could even practice with them and they could tell you whether or not it sounds good. Just be careful, especially if you're in a committed relationship. This might be edging the line a bit.

Idea: If you call and just get their voicemail, leave them a breathy message telling them how much you're thinking about them. If you really want to go bold and get really naughty, masturbate over the phone. They'll be fantasizing on how to recreate these sounds later.

Video Chat

Thanks to the wonderful inventions of things like Skype and FaceTime, video chat sex has become popular among partners long distance (or otherwise). It makes sense; it's an easy way to actually see your partner face to face. It's a new concept, so a lot of people are pretty anxious about trying it. Unlike with phone sex or sexting, and similar to real time, face to face dirty talk, it instantaneous and can be difficult coming up with what to say and it can be awkward at times.

It's similar to dirty talking in that yes, you should spend a bit of time getting pumped up for the main event. Foreplay is still important. Compliment them on how they look. On your side, make sure you put some effort into how you look. A sexy striptease on camera is never a bad thing.

You also need to prep your space just like you would if they were actually coming over. Sexting and phone sex are not visual, but video chat sex is. Pick up your clothes, make your bed, make sure there isn't garbage everywhere. It can totally turn your partner off if all they can see in the background is how messy your place is.

Sex toys are not a bad thing for investing in. Direct your partner how to use them on screen, and vice versa. There are even sex toys that come with their own apps and can be controlled from thousands of miles away. But they can be pricey, so seriously consider that before you make an investment.

Pen and Paper

People really underestimate the value of writing things down. In a world full of social media and instant messaging, it can be really special to receive a letter in the mail, especially handwritten ones. It's a lost art that deserves to be found again. It can also come off as a total surprise and very unexpected. Think about it. When's the last time you received an actual handwritten letter in the mail?

Letters are a solid thing that can be felt and be read over and over again. You don't have to send your partner a long, sappy love letter, but you can definitely light the fire in your life with just some black ink and a card. Some of these can absolutely be done over email, too, so if that's your thing, don't worry about it.
But, if you are going to send your partner some sexy notes, here are a few things to keep in mind.

Keep your handwriting neat, and if you're going to do cursive, make sure it's readable. The last thing you want to do is write a note or letter for your partner and have them being unable to read it. That could be awkward.

No issues with rough drafts. Everyone has been there when you're writing a text or email to someone you like and you just can't get it right, so you write it over and over and over again until you get it perfect. There's no shame in starting over a few times. The nice thing about sending notes and letters, rather than texting, is that you don't have to think on your feet quite as fast. The mood can't be broken so easily.

Use a lot of descriptive words. You probably already know the recipient of your notes or letters fairly well, so it shouldn't be too hard to come up with some things you want to tell them. Really spend a few days focusing on them and look for what you want to write about. Talk about how they move, how they smell, how hot they look. Really use these descriptive words. Some memorable adjectives to use include: deep, wicked, hot, spicy, dirty, insatiable, addictive, etc. If you really want to make it personal, use the ones you know they like or describe them explicitly.

Write about how they make you feel. If your goal is to be especially naughty, so what actions do they make you want to do? Words like taste, arouse, tempt, tremble, hunger, attack, pounce, devour, excite and tremble are all viable options. Write about how when you see them, you feel like you're going to explode from wanting them so bad. Or you're so tempted to just rip their clothes off, they're so hot.

Finally, write about what you want to do to them. Take the description, and the action, and put them together. Write about what you plan on doing to them, or what you wish you could do. Everything you write should be non-threatening and flattering, and especially focus on how much you want to please them.

Don't forget to write on the level of intimacy and commitment you share with this person. If you're unsure, don't put it in there. You should also avoid mentioning big words like love. This includes over text or email.

Here are just a few ways you use these tips. Even people who don't consider themselves very wordy shouldn't have too much trouble with these.

1) Send your partner a gift and write a sexy note to go with it. Send your lady flowers and write a sexy note in the card about her "other flower", wink wink. Send your man a can of whipped cream or chocolate syrup and write how you want to lick it off him later. If you want to get really raunchy, send your panties or your boxers, and make a point to point out that you'll have nothing underneath when you see each other again. Just make sure that no one else sees it, especially if they're at work. Getting fired would ruin the mood.
2) Next time you're at a restaurant together, write a quick, sexy note on a napkin and slide it across the table to them. Watch their reaction and just smile as innocently as you can. Exchange notes the entire time you're there if you're up for it. Just don't let the waiter see or that could be an awkward dinner.
3) Play "sexy pen pals". We all know what a pen pal is, right? You might have even had one as a kid. Write letters to your partner, actual letters, like you are complete strangers writing

from far away to each other. This is great if you're long distance, as you can actually act out the fantasies when you see each other. Even if you're not long distance, this can be hot where the two of you just exchange letters (or emails) and you never mention them outside of it. Describe fantasies, sexual escapades, and ask each other sexy questions. It could lead to role play where you act as if this is your first time meeting at a hotel.

4) Exchange notes. If long letters and emails just aren't your thing, just write notes. Leave a note at their work and get someone, like a secretary or assistant, to deliver it (make sure no one sees what's inside!). Buy a pack of sticky notes and put up reminders all over your partner's home where you know only they will see them. Pack their lunch and put it in there. Stick it to their bathroom mirror or on their alarm clock. Play a game of "Finish the Fantasy" using only your sticky notes (see Chapter 8 on games you can play in the bedroom).
5) Write down a fantasy in the style of an erotic story. This can be done over email or through letters. You can even just write it down and leave it somewhere you know they'll find it, especially, if you're going to be gone for a few days. You could also pack it in their suitcase or briefcase if they're going to be the ones going to be gone. Tip: Sprinkle a little cologne or perfume over it so you know it smells of you. As

they're reading it, they'll definitely be thinking of you. When you get together, you can even read it out to each other.

6) Make a "sex menu". Get out your colored pencils and use your creativity to write up what's on the menu for that night, and send it to them. Just like reading the menu before heading to a restaurant and thinking of what they want to order, you'll be the only thing on their mind. Bonus points if you tell them to pick an appetizer, a main course, and a dessert and you're ready and waiting for them to come and see you. This is a great way to add some variety to the bedroom, and because you'll only be writing out things you'll be willing to try, and they'll be picking, you'll be one hundred percent certain it's something they want.
7) Write down a list of all the things you think make a great time in the bedroom. Think "Passion", "foreplay", and "you". Send them the list and encourage them to make their own. You can exchange them and go over them together.
8) Write a sexy poem. Write a haiku. They're easy to do, even for people who consider themselves terrible at poetry. It's three lines: The first line has five syllables, the second has seven, and the last has five. Really easy. Another idea is to take all the letters of the alphabet or their name, and for every letter, write a word that starts with that letter describing what you want to do to them or how sexy they are. Or, just google some sexy poetry. A quick web search of

“sexy poetry” will show up hundreds of thousands of results. Google is your friend!

Here are some sexy ideas for notes, or even some things to get your creative juices flowing. Whether you’re looking for something poetic, sensual, funny, or dirty, you’ll find something that fits perfectly for you and your partner.

- Your lips are like honey. Your kisses are like wine.
- I love the way you explore my body with your hands.
- You’re an ideal woman! In public, you are an ice queen, but for me, you become my naughty girl.
- I get horny each time I see you, and it’s all your fault. You’re so hot.
- I love everything about you except for your clothes. Take them off.
- If you have a rough day, I’ll always be there to give you a rough night.
- You’re so hot.
- I’ve been thinking about you naked all day.
- The most productive thing I’ve done all day is thinking about you naked. Happy now?
- You can have me any way you want.

All in all, sexting, video chat, phone sex and through the mail, they're all really just other kinds of dirty talk, and very similar with a few key differences. All of these can add to your sex life, or maybe just one or two. Maybe, you're just not into it at all. That's completely fine.

Chapter 5: Upping the Pressure

Eventually, you're going to want to find yourself wanting to up the intensity. While we've talked a lot about some easy, basic things you can do to get started inside the bedroom, you could find yourself getting curious. When you get more comfortable with the idea of dirty talk, it might be time to move out of your comfort zone.

This is when you get more hardcore.

Hardcore fantasies can be difficult to explain to your partner. They require hardcore words, a lot of open-mindedness, and trust in your partner. Being wild, inhibited and completely comfortable with your partner will make things more exciting. It will bring more new things into your bedroom, some of them you've thought about for a long time and others that you've never thought about but enjoy.

Really remember your vocabulary. Your words are your greatest weapons when it comes to dirty talk, and even more when you're really getting into the more hardcore fantasies.

Go back and watch some porn. Really try stuff that you haven't ever thought of before. Note all your triggers, what gets you going, and what is a hard no. You could even watch it with your partner and keep track of their reactions.

Don't forget the erotic novels, as well. If there was a story that you thought was too intense and a bit much at the start, how do you feel about them now that you've been getting a bit naughty?

Really bring your partner into this. Challenge each other. Play some of the games mentioned in chapter 8 on role play. There's an entire section on sexy and X-rated fun to try!

Think about some of the surprises you've encountered over your dirty talk journey. Maybe, your partner has referred to you in a derogatory way, like "bastard" or "bitch" which you would have hated outside the bedroom, but you really liked. It's all about context, babe.

Here are some phrases to look over and think about. How do you feel about them?

- I love your d***/p****.
- Your ____ is perfect for my ______.

- Give it to me, you sexy bitch/bastard.
- F*** me harder.
- You want that, don't you, you slut?
- You like it when I f*** you, don't you? Tell me.
- I want you on your knees, sucking out my c***/p****
- F*** me. Right now.
- I'm so f******* wet for your c***/I'm so f****** hard for your p****.

The more you get into dirty talk, you might find yourself thinking of things that you definitely would not be touching with a ten-foot pole before. This is normal. All it means is you're becoming more sexually open-minded and adventurous. Your sexual comfort zone is widening, and baby, you're soaring.

Dirty Talking in Public

While dirty talking in public might not necessarily be considered hardcore, it can be daunting and a bit awkward. Up until now, dirty talk has mostly just been between you and your partner. But if you have a love of showing off and get off on the idea of getting caught, dirty talking in public could be right up your alley. Lust has no bounds, and you could be feeling it at a public park, the middle of a department store, the library, or the pool.

It could literally be done anywhere, in front of everyone. The only trick is that nobody knows exactly what you're thinking, and it becomes a sexy secret just between you and your partner. If you can get them pumped up and ready in a public setting, imagine the fireworks when you're in private.

Some quick tips to get started:

- Whisper it. Or at least make sure nobody can hear you. There's something super sexy about the wildest, raunchiest thing you can think of being said in a sultry whisper. Say what you want to do to them, or what you want them to do to you. Even just something like "I want to rip that shirt off of you" could be enough to get the mood going.
- Show it. Remember how you read that body language matters? Well, if you're in a situation where you can't be really explicit with your mouth, use your eyes and hands. Look at your partner's tight ass. Be coy with your eyes. Put your arm around them. Squeeze an inappropriate place for just a second, before anyone else notices.
- Take advantage of times you are alone. Pull them aside for just a few moments in a secluded spot and get a bit hot and heavy. Not so long that someone notices you're gone, but long enough that the message gets across.

- Double entendres. Something that can come off as totally innocent to the people surrounding you can come off as extremely hot to your partner. Once they get the idea in their head the most innocent of the things you say can come off as extremely dirty. You could even make it a game where you tell them at the beginning of the night you'll be making some dirty talking, and they could keep count. Example: Someone could be complaining about how hot it is, and you could whisper in your partner's ear: "we could make it hotter if you want."

Here are some good examples:

- "I can't wait to get you home and naked."
- "I bet that shirt of yours looks so much better on the floor." They will immediately start thinking about you with your clothes on the floor.
- "What a sweet, sexy ass. I'm going to put it to good use." First, you pay a compliment. Then you allude that something's going to be going down that night.
- "I want you so bad."

Chapter 6: Dirty Talk for Her

One of the most common, and ridiculous, notion about women and sex is that women don't like dirty talk. This is crazy. There is no shortage of women who like dirty talk or who are, at least, curious to try it out.

Why does this notion exist? Well, society strikes again!

There is enormous societal pressure for women. They're often featured as delicate flowers who shouldn't be sullied by dirty things. They're encouraged to keep their sexuality hidden and those who don't are shamed. This includes things like sexual expression, experimentation, porn, and discovery. It's a grim reminder of times when a woman's value was measured by her virginity or her marriage.

Now, things are different and much better. It's not the best it could be, but we're getting there. More and more women are getting in touch with their sexual identity, and more and more women are getting more confident in what they want. Women are now more openly encouraged to explore these things and take time to think about them. Times have changed, for the better. Believe it or not, studies actually show that women are more likely to indulge in sexual experimentation at some point in their lives when in comparison to men!

Of course, there are people out there who say that dirty talk is demeaning to women. They should only be getting warm, gentle, and loving words from their partner. If this is your thing, by all means, go for it, but not every woman wants that. It again goes back to women being "delicate flowers" who require a soft and gentle touch. Dirty talk is not demeaning. It actually helps women become more confident, rather than knocking them down.

Yes, women like dirty talk, and it works. A well-timed, well thought out phrase will get your woman climbing you like a tree if you do it right.

Women Like Dirty Talk But...

Keep in mind that women are pickier when it comes to the why, when, where, and who of dirty talk. Women tend not to appreciate a guy leering at her from across the club or whistling at her from across the street, especially one she doesn't know. Most of this has to do with our society's expectations on women, and sexism, but that's for another book. But the most important thing to learn is the why, when, where, and who part of the equation.

How do you figure out the why, when, where, and who? Well, it can be a bit tricky. It really varies from woman to woman. Every woman is different, and every woman will like different things. It's all about knowing your lady, and there's a good chance that she might already know what she likes. Because women are more prone to experimentation when compared to men, they might already have experienced dirty talk. So, make sure you ask them what they like. They will tell you.

Just remember, if you expect open-mindedness from her, you should be doing it yourself. It's a two-way street.

Why Women Like Dirty Talk

This is where it goes into the psychology of men versus women.

Unlike with men, who for the most part know exactly what they like, women tend to react sexually to a much larger variety of things. According to a theory, women become wet at any hint of sexual activity, but, but, wait for it, this response doesn't necessarily reflect their inner desires. So, just because a woman can have sex, that doesn't mean she actually wants to. This comes down to why dirty talk is so important: it's a way of getting her mind around to the idea of sex.

Women like foreplay. That's it. Dirty talk, being the most versatile of all foreplay, can start at any time of the day, and more importantly, it actually shows you're thinking of her. Women need to know you find them attractive, and they need to know you're thinking of them. Women love words and like to visualize. They think about what they mean and really mull over them. They will think about how their partner will react, imagine the sensations of certain things and wonder about the next time they see their partner.

Yes, telling them a few times before sex that you find them hot is great. It probably works. But letting them know just how sexy you find them as you walk out the door? Sending them a text saying you're thinking of them in the middle of the day? Actions speak louder than words, and your lady will notice. Five minutes a day, every day, goes a long way.

So, what kind of dirty talk do women generally like?

Again, every woman is different. There is no one way a woman likes to be made love to, just like there is no one way a woman likes to be dirty talked to. There is no one way to do this.

The easiest way to find out what your lady likes is to really just ask her. Finding out what your partner likes and dislikes is important, just as it's important they find out yours.

Some women like being called degrading terms like "slut" or "whore", while others hate that. Others enjoy being more submissive, while others more dominant. Some women like both. Some women like role play, while others prefer to avoid it. But, if you can find a woman out there who doesn't enjoy being told how sexy she is, well, she's definitely one of a kind.

One thing you absolutely have do is make sure you sound genuine. Make sure you're paying attention to what you're saying and that's coming out of your mouth. If it doesn't sound genuine, your lady will know it.

Be sexy. This instruction is kind of vague, but here's an easy way to look at it; just focus on all of the stuff you shouldn't be. Don't be too aggressive, insensitive, awkward, or creepy.

Aggression is about finding the right balance; too much and your woman might actually find you threatening, and too little and she won't be feeling anything at all; she just won't notice you. Don't just jump straight into the sexy talk without preparing your woman for it. Aggression means being the one to lead and not being scared

to do so. If you find yourself getting too aggressive, try behaving more playful and fun. It will help her feel at ease, and men who know how to have fun and make women laugh are sexy to women. What's not sexy is a man whose entire being seems to be based around getting into a woman's pants.
Insensitivity. Insensitivity is when you're at your partner's grandpa's funeral and you think that this is the right time to joke about how this is the first time he's been stiff in 20 years. It's all about knowing what to say at a certain time. It's like this; if your lady has had a bad day and wants to talk to you about it, right as she's in the middle of telling you how her boss chewed her out is not the time to make a move. If you do end up doing this, just try to rub it off as you couldn't resist her, and that you've been thinking about it all day. She just might melt and forget about it.

Awkwardness. Awkwardness naturally follows insensitivity, and then creepiness. When you say the wrong thing, it kills the mood and you might find yourself both just not wanting to get down and dirty.

Finally, being creepy. Creepiness is an interesting one because it is a problem a lot of men have. They often say things or do things that are meant to come off as sexy or sweet or funny and they just make a woman's skin crawl. Things like staring at her for a long period of time, acting really nervous, acting arrogant, not reading into signals, all these things can be seen as creepy.

Always, always, always remember who you're talking to. If it's your girlfriend, your wife, or long-term partner, they're going to remember the things you say. Talk to her beforehand on words she likes and doesn't like (and tell her the words you don't like and like as well) and remember the context. For example, just calling her "slut" might send some wrong messages, but "sexy slut" or "horny slut" can come off as really, really hot.

Some Phrases for You and Your Lady:

- "You are a nonstop c*** tease."
- "Smart and sexy. You're lethal."
- "Every single one of your curves deserves to be worshipped."
- "Do you even notice everyone checking you out?"
- "You're so hot."
- "I'm picturing you naked. Right now."
- "You have no idea what I'm going to do to you tonight. And you're going to like it." Their brains will immediately start to race with all of the things they have to look forward to.

- “Feel how ready I am for you.” Whisper this in her ear and press yourself up against her so she can feel exactly how ready you are. This will have her shaking in anticipation.”

Chapter 7: Dirty Talk for Him

Ever heard the saying "a man wants a lady in the streets and a hoe in the sheets"?

While this idea is pretty ridiculous, it's kind of true. Men like to have women who are open-minded and kinky in the bedroom, while not giving a hint of that side of themselves around anyone else but them.

Men want to know that you're really into him, and one way you can do this is dirty talk.

Men Like Dirty Talk But...

Men are not nearly as picky as women when it comes to why, when, where, and who. Men are always ready for sex. Contrary to the popular myth, they don't think about sex all the time, but they definitely think about it more often than women. Especially when sex is thrown in society's face all the time, whether it's the sexy image of a woman on a magazine or a sex scene in a film. But, while women like to visualize, men like to hear.

One of the biggest complaints men have about women is the fact that they're too quiet in bed. They want to hear you moaning, whimpering, screaming, sighing, and most importantly, they want to know that they're doing the right thing. They want to know that their partner is enjoying themselves, and you squirming, moaning, and begging for more is really what's going to do it for them.

Society tends to portray men as having to be the best of the best of the best, and they must always be the "alpha male". It's a popular trope in fiction; the sexy, bulky with arm muscles for days man gets the girl while his usually geeky friend with the glasses gets usually nobody. The sexy, alpha male is the leader, the protector, and the provider. Men want to feel this way in real life. You can help make him feel that way.

This comes back to our primal needs and wants. Men like to dominate. They like to be wanted. They want to know just how much their woman is into them. There have, actually, been studies on the fact that while women want to be pleasured, men want to be the ones doing the pleasuring. Meaning, they get excited about the idea of bringing their partner to ecstasy.

While this may not be true in every man, and just like women, men like a variety of different things in their sex life. No two men will like all exactly the same things. Men also tend to know what they like, and they want to stick with it. By a certain age (somewhere in their 20s), they have likely done most of the experimentation they will ever do. So knowing what your man likes is always really important.

Men do actually want to communicate. They might not be that good at it at times, but they want to. They want to make things better, for you and for them. A man who cares about your wants and needs will make the time if that's what you need. If they don't, well, they're an ass.

Why Men Like Dirty Talk

Don't underestimate compliments. Men love compliments; they just don't hear them often. While women will often spend hours complimenting their friend's hair, their makeup, their manicure, men just don't get this. Men don't compliment other men.

So, when a woman compliments a man, it gives him a confidence booster. It lets him know that he's doing something right, that he's the best in the world. OK, maybe not the best in the world. Being genuine is important, just like it is for women, and reminding your man just how much you find him attractive in a way that's personal gets you bonus points. Men don't get romanticized nearly as much as women do, which is a shame; because men are sexy and gorgeous too!

Men need confidence boosters just as much as women do. So, when you're talking dirty with your man, really focus on how sexy you find them and how amazing they're doing. How hot he is. How much he turns you on. He's a stallion! But, do be honest and genuine, especially if you're in the middle of the deed or you're referring to a specific part of them. Men will catch on if you're not telling the truth, because, yes, they need the confidence booster, they also need to know what exactly it is about them that gets you hot.

Bo bold. While men need confidence boosters, they also want to know they're with a confident woman who knows what they want. Going after what you want and knowing exactly what it is is a good thing.

Don't fake anything. If you're not feeling anything, *don't fake it.* No matter what you do. This does not make things good for you, your partner, or any future partner they have. If they think they're doing it right for you, they'll keep doing it. You'll keep being unsatisfied, and they'll keep thinking they're doing a good thing. Nobody wins in this scenario.

Some Phrases to Get Your Man All Hot:

- "Do you think I have panties on right now?" Anything relating to your underwear, or lack of underwear, will get him going.
- "If you keep looking at me that way, I'm not responsible for what happens to your c***." His imagination will run wild. You know exactly where.
- "Get over here." Forward, and to the point.
- "I can't imagine sharing you with anyone." Yes, too much possessiveness is a bad thing. But a little bit is a good thing. It's healthy.
- "Just looking at you makes me wet." Anything to remind him how hot you find him.
- "You feel so good, baby." Seriously, anything.
- "I want you between my legs, right now."

Chapter 8: Some X Rated Games

Sex is supposed to be fun. It may be for adults, but there's no reason you can't act like a little kid. Play away some fun games or some role play!

Role Play

Dirty talking is often considered a stepping stone into role play. While dirty talk is all about telling a story to your partner and turning them on by putting images into their mind, roleplaying is about actually acting out the fantasy.

Eventually, you're probably going to want to try it out. And for good reason! It's fun. At this point, you and your partner have probably, actually shared some fantasies with each other and talked openly about things you want to try in the bedroom. If you have a fantasy that the two of you share, this is a perfect play to start off with.

Once you've started really getting into role play, there's an entire world out there dedicated to it - books, podcasts, websites, online communities. They'll have ideas and suggestions on what to do and how to make it better. While you'll likely find some things that make you pause, you might find one or two fantasies that you've never even considered but now definitely want to try.

Of course, role-playing can be nerve-wracking, kind of weird, at least the first few times, and a bit terrifying. Roleplaying is often built on fantasies, either yours or your partner's, and that's the really scary part. Sharing your fantasies with your partner can make you nervous because you're sharing one of your innermost desires. You don't know what their reaction will be. Will they laugh at you? Will they think you're a freak? Will they love the idea or hate it?

If telling your partner makes you anxious, the actual act can make someone lose their mind even more. What if one of you breaks character and the mood is totally broken? What if one of you messes up and someone gets hurt? What if you end up really liking it and they hate it so much that they never want to do it again?

Yes, the idea of role play can turn you into a pile of nervous jello, but it can also be fun, liberating, and most importantly, sexy. It's like playing imagination games like a kid only they're X-rated.

As we grow up, we're encouraged to shut down that side of ourselves. We see it as "silly" and "childish." We get embarrassed by the thought. But kids don't worry about it, and neither should you. Letting your imagination and creativity run wild is not a bad thing, and definitely should not be stamped out. Let it roam!

Here are some tips to get you started.

Steps to Take

First: What is your fantasy? This seems pretty obvious, but it's important. You need to figure out what you like. Don't worry too much about whether or not your partner will like it in this step, because this is strictly for you. It can be super cheesy or porny as you'd like. Maybe it relates to your life, such as your job or the TV shows you're watching or something from your past. For example, a lot of people who have ever had a crush on one of their college professors have fantasized about the naughty student scenario. Yes, it's cliché, but if you think it's hot, go for it. If you're really not coming up with anything, you can always try watching your favorite porn.

Second: Tell your partner. If you really want this to happen, this step is unavoidable. You're going to need to get comfortable with telling your partner about your fantasies first, of course, but if you've never done it before, you can try saying something like; "I had such a hot dream about you last night". They'll likely ask, and you can go into details. Even if you didn't have a dream, it's an easy step to take. You can also email or text it if you're more comfortable that way. If it relates to a TV show, talk about it while you're watching the show. Of course, at some point, you're going to have to tell them why you're telling them, and you want to roleplay it. But be warned; you're going to have to be really specific as to why this scenario turns you on. Maybe, you like the masseuse-client fantasy, but you like the masseuse to be really passionate and desperate for more, and the power dynamic gets you going.

Third: Set some boundaries. This is an important step because you don't want to be halfway into it and one of you goes too far. This is especially important if you're acting out a scenario that involves punishment. Talk it out, and figure out what you want. This is especially important if one of you has triggers or words you don't like. Maybe, you want to act out a hot scene from a show, but dislike the nicknames the characters call each other. Maybe you're a sexy maid or butler that needs to be punished, but you want a light spanking, and hate the idea of waking up with a handprint-shaped bruise on your butt. Safe words are never a bad idea.

Fourth: Set the scene. Wardrobe definitely isn't mandatory, but it's a whole lotta fun. Things like wigs, a frilly apron, a cape, body oil, all these things add to the experience and really get you into your roles. Same goes for the where. No, you can't turn your bedroom into a 15th century themed brothel house, but lighting some candles and hanging up some curtains goes a long way.

Fifth: HAVE FUN. Don't worry too much about whether or not one of you breaks character. If something doesn't work out, it doesn't work out. If your partner ends up not enjoying something, then they can just use the safe word, and vice versa. The aim is the feel turned on, not get a role in a Hollywood film. Remember what you read about how as adults we're supposed to leave playing with our imagination behind? With roleplaying, you don't have to leave it in the past. Your first time might make you feel a little nervous, but that's normal. Just go for it and have a good time!

Some Roleplaying Ideas

Just in case you're running a bit blank, here's a quick list of some roleplaying ideas. Which ones do you it for you?

1) Repairman/woman. Maybe your kitchen is broken and you have no way to pay them. If you really want to get it, get the person doing the repairing actually drive up into the house wearing overalls or flannel, while the other can answer the door wearing almost nothing. You can go through an entire

thing where the repairperson takes off their clothes because of how “hot” it’s getting.

2) Student-Teacher. Anybody who had a hot professor in college can relate. The variations to this one are endless. Are you working at a public school? A private school? What kind of class is it? Is the student a teacher’s pet or a rebel?
3) Stripper. One of you can give the other a lap dance. Bring in some dollar bills if you really want to get into it. Choose a sexy song, consider wearing body glitter or cover your chest with body oil to make it glisten, dim the lights for ambiance, and pick a stripper name like Jasmine or Dominick, and go wild.
4) Strangers at a bar. Both of you dress up (don’t let the other person see you before you go), go to a hotel or bar separately, and “meet” up there. You can make up your own names, your jobs, whatever you want! You could even recreate the first time you met.
5) Favorite movie/TV Show. I’m sure one of you has a favorite sex scene in a film and thinks it’s the hottest thing ever. Or choose an iconic couple from a TV series and roll with it. Ross and Rachel, anyone? Think of iconic lines or scenes and try to recreate it.
6) Prostitute. Call in your partner, and “hire” them to do whatever you want to them. Get as over the top and fake as you want.

7) Masseuse. Break out the body oil, light some candles, and really get into it. Bonus; you get a massage. Set it up so the two of you are dressed minimally. Shirtless massages are the best massages.
8) Favorite celebrity couple. Beyoncé and Jay-Z? Angelina Jolie and Brad Pitt? Kim and Kanye? Elizabeth Taylor and Richard Burton? The choice is yours. Google the couple of your choosing, and try to mimic their style or tone of speaking. Watching YouTube videos of them speaking could help. If they have nicknames for each other, use these too.
9) Server-Customer. Anything customer service related goes, really. Set the table with a tablecloth and candlesticks. The server can wear a button-down shirt and black slacks and the customer can wear their best dress.
10) Royalty. Anyone who was obsessed with Disney movies growing up would enjoy this role play. Pick a princess or prince you want to try out. You could order really extravagant costumes online or even just wear a wig. It doesn't necessarily have to be make-believe royalty; there's no shame in playing Harry and Meghan!
11) Doctor and Nurse. Cliché? Yes. Hot? Oh yeah, babe. Wear white uniforms, unless you decide to go for surgeon's scrubs instead. You could use stethoscopes, clipboards, and gloves. You could examine your patient, ask questions, and give sponge baths.

12) Boss-Employee. Anyone who has ever had a super cute boss will understand. The boss can call the employee in to have a talk about their performance, or try to debate a raise. Just like teacher-student, there are a ton of possibilities. Wear professional clothing and really try to recreate that work setting.
13) Cheerleader, football captain. While you could get authentic costumes from thrift stores or online or even your own high school closet, they're not hard to recreate. Football players have jerseys who can be sexy jerks who constantly get down in the locker room or nervous virgins new to the team. Cheerleaders keep their hair in ponytails, carry pompoms, and wear short skirts and crop tops, and can be angelic virgins who wear a promise ring or can be sleeping with the entire football team, and even some cheerleaders.
14) Hero. Take your pick. Firefights, superheroes, romantic citizens carry you out of buildings and push you out the front of heavy buildings. They save you, then lovingly give you medical treatment including massage, bathing, and sex. If you decide to go the superhero route, you could try one that you wanted to be real when you were a kid. It will add an element of excitement.

The roleplaying ideas really are endless, and all the variations make the list ten to twenty times longer. Mix and match on what you want to do. You could try every single one you've ever even heard of and there would still be more to try out there.

But for beginners, really pick something simple. It should be something that doesn't require too much preparation, with minimal props and something one of you is at least a little familiar with. If you're playing a cop, pick up some toy handcuffs, a badge, and a plastic gun. Adopt a stern demeanor and get ready to make some sexy arrests. Really take the time to get into your character.
Look on the internet or your local sex store for props. Some will be pretty easy to find, like a sexy maid outfit, while others may take some digging. If you want to go all out, you can. But you can still have fun as a sexy maid with just the frilly apron. You don't really need the whole get up. And, it can be costly.

Ask yourself questions about the act you're playing. How does the role behave? Are they a nervous, inexperienced virgin or a horny slut who just wants to get off? Is their behavior an act, or is this how they're always in and out of the bedroom? If it makes it easier, try to relate your real-life emotions to the character. Or use a scenario you've experienced in real life.

Always remember your motivation, and why you're doing this; because you want to get turned on. You want the two of you to have a good, exciting time. Is this also your character's goal? Or is it something different? Often, the goal of the character is to humiliate, embarrass, or punish your partner. Remember that.

Don't forget the dirty talk to go along with it! The whole point is to turn the heat up and get the engines running. Keep the sexy times rolling, and keep it in line with what you're trying to accomplish. For example, a dirty cop might allude to how bad the criminal has been, or do a sexy pat down, going as far as to fondle them up a bit. You can get very creative, trying to keep the dirty talk on topic, but this kind of dedication only ups the intensity and makes it better. This can, of course, eventually turn into a lifestyle. There are people out there whose entire relationship is built around role play, and BDSM. But, whether it's just something you indulge in occasionally or a regular occurrence in your bedroom, it's a hell lotta fun.

Sex Games

Games are great. Games are fun. Sex is great. Sex is fun. Why shouldn't they mix? Sex games aren't technically dirty talk, but they can be a fun way of communicating and trying new things. They are also a great way to get into dirty talk and make yourself more comfortable at the idea of talking about sex with your partner.

Oldies but Goodies:

1) Sexy truth or dare. Take two containers, one for truths and one for dares. Write on slips of paper the truths and dares. Take turns asking each other truth or dare.

Some ideas for truths: What's your biggest and naughtiest fantasy? What is #1 on your sexual bucket list right now? When was the first time you pictured me naked?
Some ideas for dares: Whisper something in my ear that you think will turn me on. Show me the sexiest picture you have on your phone. Put whipped cream on a body part you want me to lick it off of. Do your best to make me orgasm in the next 5 minutes.

2) Literally, bet on anything. Play a game of strip poker. Have a contest to see who can get the most paper balls in the trash from a certain distance or angle. Play pool. Great for people who have competitive sides. Bet things like sexual acts or pieces of clothing.
3) Dice. Grab some dice, and assign each number an action. Take turns rolling, and use this guide as an example (or make up your own). You could also have one die represent a body part and another die represent an action. Mix and match!

   1 = kiss your partner's body choice their choosing.

   2 = take off one article of clothing of your partner's choosing.

   3 = kiss your partner for 1 minute.

   4 = Tell your most elaborate fantasy, and don't skimp on the details.

   5 = Kiss your partner. Where you kiss them is there choice.

6 = Do some heavy petting on your favorite part of your partner's body.

Another dice game includes strip dice, where each number represents an article of clothing to removed.

Wordplay Games

If the two of you are really into words, they'll be something here for you.

1) Play X-rated scrabble. You're only allowed to use the words that you know will get you and your partner hot and horny.
2) Play a word association game. You say a word, and your partner replies with the first thing they think of. You say "butt", your partner says "squeeze". You say "dick", your partner says "suck." See the pattern?
3) Make a dirty crossword puzzle. There are easy to find crossword puzzles to use online, and they're pretty simple to use. Put one together and give it to your partner to do over breakfast. Everyone has tried to do a crossword puzzle, right?
4) Play "finish the fantasy". The game is simple. You start off a fantasy and stop after one or two lines. Your partner picks up and makes up one or two lines. Repeat cycle. Recreate the fantasy later.
5) Rate your partner. Write out a list of sexual acts, like oral, kissing, etc., and "rate" how good your partner is. Keep in

mind, only do this if you really feel you can handle hearing that you're not a perfect 10. Be open to getting feedback and improving. If you can't do this, don't play. It will only start a fight.

Chapter 9: You and Dirty Talk

The reason you picked up this book in the first place is likely because you feel lost. Maybe, you just have no idea where to start, no idea how to do this. Maybe, your partner requested it of you and you needed some extra encouragement.

Either way, there are some things you can do. Remember, the goal is for you to actually enjoy dirty talk. It can be fun! That's what important here, for you to *have fun*. Your partner wants you to have fun too.

What You Can Do (By Yourself)

Yes, there are things you can do without a partner to make yourself better at dirty talk and feel more confident in it. Take your time, there's no rush. But remember, actually getting into the bedroom and doing it is the best way to get better. It really comes down to one thing.

Masturbate.
Masturbating is not only a good way to get in touch with your inner sex god, but it has a ton of other benefits. Books, studies, and websites have all been devoted to explaining masturbation and it's mental and physical health benefits.

It's a giant confidence booster. If you won't have sex with you, who would? When you masturbate, you're usually thinking of a fantasy of some kind. You're thinking about someone else, whether they be your partner, your childhood crush or the entire cast of Friends wanting to have sex with you. You're thinking about how they find you hot and desirable and they want you right then and there. This ripples over into your sex life with a partner, and eventually your actual life.

It helps you relax. If you find yourself super stressed and tensed up, masturbation can have the same effects as a long massage or a nice bath. When you orgasm, your brain releases oxytocin, which in studies has shown to reduce stress hormones in the brain.

It makes your sex life better. In exploring your body, you're learning what it likes and what it doesn't like. You're getting a good idea of what you would like to see happen in the bedroom and make you more confident in what you like. When you've figured this all out, you can tell your partner where to touch you with ease without worrying about what you like. More orgasms.

It helps you stay in the game. When you're going through a dry spell or simply just not finding yourself sexually motivated, masturbation can help keep sex at the forefront of your mind. There are cases when people who haven't had sex in a long time and they just aren't thinking about it. If you're thinking about sex, you're more likely to go out there and get sex.

It can benefit your partner, too. If you're in a relationship, it's something different. Just like it's noted above, the more sex you have, the more sex you'll want. Being self-sexual will stimulate your brain and keep your libido alive and well. This will be beneficial to your partner.

Really, there are no downsides. It has absolutely zero negative side effects. It's good for your brain, your health, your sex life, and your partner. And it feels AMAZING.

But, don't just masturbate for the sake of masturbating and having an orgasm. Yes, if you're seasoned at playing with yourself, you probably just want to get it over with. You think of the orgasm as the goal. But, if you want to make your sex life better, slow is the way to go. Orgasms are great, but they're not always the goal. The goal here to get to know yourself and what you think.

Really just take the time to get to feel your body, figure out what you like and just embrace and savor every moment.
When you masturbate, think of it almost like you would pleasing a partner, only you're pleasing yourself. You could even do foreplay, where you spend the day looking at yourself in mirrors and complimenting yourself as to how hot you are. You could even masturbate in front of a mirror if you're into some experimentation.

Really think about the last time you got turned on. Think about why it turned you on. Reliving the experience can help you figure out what you like and help you control the intensity.

You shouldn't just run for the orgasms. Bring yourself to the brink, and bring yourself down again. Rotate between fast and slow. Your orgasm will be more intense the more buildup there is.

Talk dirty to yourself. Yes, you read that right. Talk yourself up. Mention how much you love it when you do something to yourself. Tell yourself how sexy you are. It may feel a little silly at first, but it works. This is a great time to figure out what kind of words you like and don't like. Narrate yourself. Really get into it. Nobody's around to hear it, why do you care?

Try out new things and really get to know what you like and don't like. What words do you like? Which ones turn you on? Are there words that turn you off? Say words you wouldn't normally say and try them out. Keep saying it, keep talking, until you find what you really like. This will really help you work up your sex vocabulary and you'll be able to go into dirty talk knowing *exactly* what you want to hear. This takes a lot of pressure off you, and your partner.

You could also try keeping a journal. Not just any journal; a sexy journal. A little black book but for a whole other reason. Keep track of what you like and don't like. Write down your fantasies. Write down the words you like. Do you have a sexy bucket list? Write it down! Keep track of the things you know your partner likes or the words they like. Anything you feel you need to write down, make sure you do. It could be fun later if you're looking for inspiration, you could read it and maybe find something you've forgotten about! You could even get your partner to keep a journal as well, and swap ideas and thoughts.

One easy exercise you can do in the journal is to really take time to reflect. Remember, learning to dirty talk is almost like learning another language. Writing things down really can help you learn to express yourself sexually and help you learn the language of love. Or dirty talking, whatever you want to call it.

Let's Talk about Fantasies

Fantasies. If you claim you've never had a fantasy in your life, well, then you're a liar. Human beings are sexual creatures, and we think about sex. It's just a fact of life. There's nothing bad about it. The world may be telling you it's bad and it's shameful, but it's not. You're going to read that, over and over again, until it sinks in. It should not be bad or shameful to have fantasies; it's healthy and normal. It's actually a large part of our biological coding.

There are people out there who will claim that fantasizing about someone else is cheating on your partner. That's ridiculous. By fantasizing, you're expressing yourself sexually and exploring the possibilities, not cheating. So, if you think that you fantasizing about your celebrity crush is a bad thing, forget it.

Asking someone not to fantasize is like asking someone not to eat. It's just not natural to expect someone not to do it. Now, whether or not they act on them is an entirely different story, but at the same time, it's not likely to actually lead to these actions. Even if the fantasy is considered wrong in real life, like incest, rape, or pedophilia, does not necessarily mean that you're going to commit these acts.

Fantasies come in huge varieties. In sex fantasies, there are definitely some forbidden topics that we only visit in our minds, but there are others that can make a reappearance again and again. Revisit them until you are comfortable to share them if you're up for it. Keep in mind that some fantasies just should not be shared. If you know it's something that would make your partner angry or uncomfortable and put a strain on the relationship, keep it to yourself for your own enjoyment.

Confidence

Confidence is important. You need to be sure of your abilities to turn your partner on and keep them in the mood. They should be doing the same for you. It's a two-way street, so you need to be doing your part!

Some tips on building your confidence are:

1) Compare yourself to others? Just don't. Nothing kills your confidence faster quite like comparing yourself to others. If you're first getting into dirty talk, but your partner has done it quite a bit before, don't obsess over comparing yourself to their former partner. Don't think about it. But if you must, just remember; their old partner would've had a first time

too, and likely felt just as insecure and uncomfortable as you are.

2) Make sure you're comfortable. Your first time trying dirty talk is going to feel awkward and like you're out of place. You're going to wish that the floor would just swallow you up. That's very normal. Your first time trying dirty talk, try to do it with someone with whom you're okay with looking silly in front of, or at least in a place that's safe for you.
3) Look your best. Wear some nice clothes. Shave wherever you feel you need to or don't shave if you feel you don't need to. Work out. Eat healthily. Constantly worrying about your appearance makes it difficult for you to put yourself out there. Taking these steps will help, and the health benefits are great too.
4) Don't think about failure. Failure is the number one reason why people don't want to try new things. They think they won't like it, they'll look like an idiot, or they will come out unsatisfied and feeling like they just wasted their time. Don't worry too much about it. You won't know until you try, and even if you do fail, you can always try again. It's likely that you and your partner will eventually just have a funny story to tell.
5) Fake it, till you make it. Worst comes to worst, use some phrases from this book and just pretend to be really confident in your ability. Confidence is a learned skill, and sometimes

the best way to be confident is to just pretend you are. The more you pretend, the easier it will get. As a result, you will become more naturally confident.

Be Comfortable

Comfort is important when trying anything new sexually. You need to be with a person who you trust, and you need to be in a position that you comfortable in. Maybe you're the kind of person who can get comfortable in just a few minutes, but maybe you're not. Either one is fine.

Either way, it's important that you're relaxed. If you are completely stressed out and stiff, you're not going to have a good time. Neither is your partner because they're going to notice. Sex and dirty talking can only be good if both parties are into it, so take whatever necessary steps you need to feel this way.

As you've read this book, you've probably found yourself thinking of phrases you want to say or things you want to do, but you might still be a little uncomfortable. That's OK. There are ways you can fix that.

Try this: Pull out your sexy journal and ask yourself some questions to get you going. Here are some ideas for you:

- What's the sexiest thing you can think of?
- If you could pick out one fantasy to act out, what would it be?
- What is the one thing that turns you on more than anything else?
- Describe the last time you had sex. Was it good? What made it so good?
- Describe the hottest thing your partner has ever done.
- What's the one thing your partner can do to get you going?
- What is the one thing your partner is really, really good at?
- What do you do to get your partner going?
- Think about your partner's body. What do you love about it?
- Describe the best orgasm you ever had. What made it so great? What exactly did your partner do to get you off? Can you recreate it? (Tip: If this happened to be with your current partner, send them a copy of your description along with a thank you note.)

Is it getting hot in here or what?

But it's not just about getting comfortable with thinking the words or writing them down. You need to be comfortable with saying them, in a soft, husky voice to boot. Writing something down or talking dirty to yourself is only the first step.

There are ways to get yourself more comfortable. Yes, talking to yourself and saying things over and over again until you've really figured out what you like is great, but it's only one thing. Try talking to yourself in the mirror.

The best advice you'll get is to really try to get all the giggles and the awkwardness out now. If you giggle every time you say the word "pussy" or "ass" just to yourself in the mirror, you might be in trouble when you come to face to face with your partner. The more comfortable you are saying these naughty words out loud the better you'll be when you actually say it to your partner. Weirdly enough, you need to get to a place where you just don't get bothered by the words anymore, at least not in an awkward way.

If it's your voice that's making your balk out of dirty talk, try using the voice recording app on your phone. Tape yourself masturbating. Again, nobody else is there, why feel awkward? Really listen to how your voice gets breathy, the sounds you make, how you feel when you hear them. Don't worry too much about mimicking it; you shouldn't have too hard a time if your partner is doing what they're supposed to. Although, you could use this as another way to figure out what you want to hear. No shame if you can get off just by the sound of your own voice; it's probably super hot!

The most important thing to remember is to never feel shame over what you want or need in the bedroom. If something turns you on, it turns you on. If it's something you can recreate with a consenting adult, great. If it's not, well, that's what your sexy journal is for!

Communication

Communication is completely underrated when it comes to sex. You need to tell your partner what gets you off, what's not working, and what is. It's baffling in this society there are a lot of people out there who don't want to or are scared to talk about it but are not enjoying sex as much as they should. Of course, this leads back to the fact that we're told our whole childhood that we shouldn't talk about sex, but details.

Partners who talk more about sex actually have better sex, believe it or not. It's a common topic of study at Universities. The gist of it is this: The more you talk about sex, the better it will be. It kind of makes sense: Dirty talk is all about communication. It's all about letting them know how much you appreciate them and how great your partner is doing. It doesn't matter how old you are or how long you've been together or even what your relationship is.

Fortunately, it's never too late to establish a better link between you and your partner. Unfortunately, some people just aren't very good at it. In a utopian world, we would learn how to communicate our wants and needs effectively and without issue, but we're not quite there yet. Bad communication is actually a very common problem, with any kind of relationship, not just sexual ones. It is usually the first thing covered in couples counseling because it's something a lot of people just don't know how to do without yelling or eyes rolling. But, like dirty talking, it is a learned skill.

First of all, you need to be comfortable. You need to be able to open up to your partner, especially if you want to try something new or it's something they or you have never done before.

Second of all, you need to give them 100 percent of your attention. No excuses. This is about you and them, and only you and them. Make sure they know you're listening. Keep eye contact. Turn off your phone.

Third of all, don't interrupt. If your partner is talking, you should be listening. Try to listen, and really think about it before you do talk. Reflect before you say anything. You should be coming in willing to listen and take suggestions.

Your partner is not a mind reader. Don't expect them to just know without actually communicating. If you don't enjoy dirty talk, let them know you'd prefer to try something else. If they're using a word you don't like, tell them the words you do like. If you want to try a hot role play involving your partner calling you "master", well, it's never going to happen unless you open your mouth.

Remember that it's give and take. Remember what if you try something for your partner, it's only right if you try something for them too. This is a common pattern in relationships: one partner does all the talking, the other just goes along with it, and it can create a pattern of resentment. Try to make sure that you're both being heard.

Communicating with your partner does not have to be a chore. It can actually be a lot of fun. People often think of communicating as two people sitting down and having a conversation about feelings, but talking about sex should be fun. After all, you're talking about new ways the two of you can enjoy yourselves, and how you can make it better for the other person.

Talk about your sexual likes and dislikes. Talk about your opinions on various role plays, scenarios, and fantasies. Discuss your views on sexuality. Plan on places to have sex. Do a sex challenge where you vow to give each other an orgasm every day for a month. Share ideas. Talk about and relive the best times the two of you have got it on. Really get down and talk about what you want from each other.

Some fun things to try include making a list of all the things you think make great sex. Think passion, excitement, role play, etc.

Another idea is to come up with a list of questions to ask each other. You could even rate each other on your various techniques, but don't do this unless you feel you could really take criticism and work on improving yourself.

Some More Phrases

- "_____ feels incredible with you." Any sex position can be used here. Use one that you actually really enjoy, because that means you're not only giving your partner an ego boost, you're guaranteeing that you'll do this position again.
- "You are going to be so sore tomorrow." The number of scenarios that are inserted into someone's mind at hearing this is breathtaking.
- "Do you want more? Beg for it." You're asking a question and telling them how to answer in one; you're dominating your control. You're showing you're the one who calls the shots.
- "Use me as your toy all night long." You're basically telling your partner "do whatever you want to me". You're showing that you trust them to put you in what could be a raw and open place without taking advantage of you, and you're welcoming them to use whatever fantasy they have to work.
- "Faster!" Say this just on the edge of when you're about to come.

- "Make me." You're practically begging for them to put you in your place!
- "You like this, don't you?" It's playful and it encourages more dirty talk. It gets your partner to engage as well.
- "I can't get enough." This tells them that you're always going to want them, no matter how long you've been together. You still want them just as much as you did the first day you had sex.
- "Come all over me."
- "Come for me." There's something so hot about hearing this, they might just cum right then and there.
- "That feels good, doesn't it?"
- "Look at me. Tell me what you see. Describe it." By getting your partner to describe the things around you, the experience will better itself for both you of you. Your brain will be stimulated hearing what they're saying, while their brains will be stimulated thanks to what they're both saying and seeing. The talking will just add to the sensory overload.

Conclusion

Thank you for making it through to the end of *How to Talk Dirty*, let's hope it was informative and able to provide you with all of the tools you need to achieve your goals, whatever they may be.

The next step is to go out there and actually talk dirty! Take these tips and jump right in and make your sex life even better! Try everything, really.

Maybe, reading this book helped you feel confident to try something new that you've never tried before. Maybe, it's validated you because you thought you were strange for not liking dirty talk. Maybe you're walking away from this book with a whole new set of ideas, thoughts, and opinions. You can't wait to try all that you've learned.

Now, you definitely want to give roleplaying a try. Now, you have the confidence to send your partner a sexy text. You want to give phone sex a shot and whisper all the naughty things you want to do with your partner in their ear while in a crowded public area. Give it a try! You won’t know exactly what you like until you actually try it.

The most important thing you can take away from this book is to have fun. Sex should be a fun experience, hands down. You should never walk away feeling not satisfied and like you didn’t get what you wanted from it. If dirty talk is the way for you to feel that way, go for it!

www.ingramcontent.com/pod-product-compliance
Lightning Source LLC
Chambersburg PA
CBHW031202050825
30641CB00034B/382

* 9 7 8 1 9 5 1 3 3 9 4 4 9 *